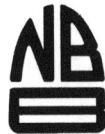

Honey for Health
Cecil Tonsley

ISBN: 978-1-912271-67-2

This publication of the original 1969 version is with
the agreement of the family of Cecil Tonsley

Published by Northern Bee Books © 2020

Northern Bee Books, Scout Bottom Farm,
Mytholmroyd, Hebden Bridge, HX7 5JS (UK)

www.northernbeebooks.co.uk

Tel: 01422 882751

Design by SiPat.co.uk

HONEY FOR HEALTH

Prehistoric man plundered the wild
bees for this valuable food.

The ancient world revered it as 'food of the gods'.
Honey from the tombs of the Pharaohs has been
found in perfect condition after thousands of
years. The Ancient Greeks believed that it would
prolong life, and in the Middle East it has been
credited with magical and aphrodisiac powers.

Its uses in medicine and surgery have led to almost
miraculous cures. Medieval man proved its healing
properties; it has cured smallpox and healed wounds.

Now in the twentieth century we are
rediscovering the wonder of honey, and
the fascination of the world of bees.

Honey for Health

Contents

Foreword... 7

Introduction... 9

Honey in History... 11

Honey in Legend and Mythology.. 17

What is Honey?.. 25

Honeys of the World.. 31

Food of the Gods.. 37

    Honey bread and cakes... 39

    Meat and poultry.. 43

    Desserts and puddings.. 54

    Honey sweets 56

    Preserves.. 58

    Additional delights.. 58

    Mead and honey drinks.. 60

Honey in Medicine and Surgery.. 67

Honey for the Children 77

Honey for Beauty.. 79

Beekeeping for Pleasure and Profit 81

Illustrations
Pages 44–53

1   The skepmaker's art. Courtesy of Eric Greenwood.
2   The beekeeper in his apiary.
3   A swarm on a tree. Courtesy of Alan Thompson.
4   'Wild' colony in a bush. Courtesy of Frederick Rath.
    Swarming bees on a skep.
5   Bee on a blackberry blossom.
6   Bee collecting nectar.
7   A comb of honey and brood from a hive. Courtesy of John Topham Ltd.
8   Bees drinking from an improvised fountain. Courtesy of R. E. Sothcott.
9   The exclusive Honey Shop in Germany.
10 The season's storehouse of honey.

Foreword

I WROTE this book on honey because I felt it was badly needed to fill a gap left since Dr Bodog Beck and Doreé Smedley's fine work *Honey and Your Health* last appeared about 1947.

I sincerely hope that this book will bring not only a better understanding of honey by the public but will also be read with pleasure, for the honey-bee is without doubt the most wonderful of all creatures to come out of the earth, and the produce of its hive has no equal as a natural food, nor are there any two products that have figured more greatly in Man's development and civilisation than honey and beeswax.

In giving thanks and acknowledgement to such works as *Honey and Your Health, The Sacred Bee, Making Mead, Old Favourite Honey Recipes, Folk Medicine*, etc., the American Honey Institute, the Australian Honey Board and to the very many friends in beekeeping who have kindly contributed to make this work possible, I am also mindful of my own inadequacies, but if when reading these pages you find enjoyment, I shall feel fully repaid.

CECIL C. TONSLEY

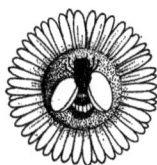

Introduction

OUR EARLIEST record of Man's interest in honey dates back to palaeolithic times. Among a series of prehistoric rock paintings discovered in 1919 at a place called Cuevas de la Arana (Spider's Cave) near Valencia, Spain, is one showing 'beekeeping', if that could be the correct term to apply to the plundering of a wild bees' nest.

In this most ancient work of art known (it was 'painted' somewhere about 15,000 years ago), two people are shown on a rudimentary rope ladder scaling a cliff. Hilda Ransome in her book *The Sacred Bee* suggested the ladder was probably made of esparto grass. The one at the top is filling a basket with combs of honey whilst warding off the fierce attack of the honey-bee owners of the nest with some smouldering material. To heighten the awesomeness of the occasion the artist has drawn the bees large in proportion to the man. The second figure appears to be mounting the ladder in readiness to receive the basket as soon as it is full of honeycomb.

The fact that prehistoric man braved the sharp stings of innumerable angry bees to obtain supplies of comb honey suggests that he must have found the stupendous effort very worthwhile and the food rewarding. So much did he value this source of food that a veneration of the honey-bee, honey and beeswax grew out of it which has continued in many parts of the world up to the present day. Even in the most civilised countries the mention of honey and the honey-bee conjures up in the mind something of this mystique, and perhaps not without some good and valid reason, as we shall see, although it is not the intention of this book to endow honey with any supernatural power.

Primitive man consumed honey in its crudest form-much as some African tribes do today—that is along with a good deal of the bee larvae and pollen combs because part of the honey-bees' food consists of pollen besides honey. He would have found the highly nutritive sweet sugars immensely satisfying and obtained protein and vitamins from both pollen and bee grubs, and also a little health-giving benefit from the beeswax comb This diet would have provided the combination of a well-filled belly and a natural medicine with gentle laxative action.

With the dawn of the first civilisations, honey became of great importance, both on medical grounds and in religious observance; honey and beeswax and the industrious bee came to be inscribed upon the records of almost every race and creed throughout the world.

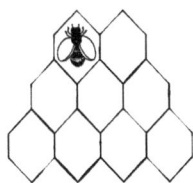

1

Honey in History

THE GREEKS had a word for it, so had the Egyptians, Assyrians, Babylonians, Romans, Hebrews and Phoenicians. From the very earliest of times honey has figured in all kinds of ceremonials, but more especially in religious and pagan worship where among the sacrifices honey would generally be found.

From Ancient Egyptian diggings and the tombs of various Pharaohs, crucibles of honey have been recovered and the honey, it is said, was as good and fragrant as the day it was sealed in with the dead king. As honey deteriorates with the passing of time in a normal atmosphere it is quite conceivable that the dry constant conditions of the great tombs of Egypt accounted for the long preservation. This was also found to be the case where honey was discovered in the caves of Crete during more recent excavations.

So important was honey to the Egyptian and his way of life that the occupation of the beekeeper is given great prominence and illustrated in the many rock pictures to be found associated with the pyramids. In these vivid illustrations the beekeeper is shown collecting honey, removing combs from the hives, straining out the particles of wax, etc., and finally sealing it in great earthenware jars for future use. Sometimes he is depicted smoking the bees to subdue them so that he can handle them quietly.

All the Middle East races laid great store by honey and believed that only through its use could one, for example, obtain eternal life or indeed enjoy the transient happiness of earth. And because the important events of living were consecrated in religious ceremonial, honey figured in rituals from birth to the grave, and it also symbolised the purity of the soul.

Egyptian bridegrooms were expected to supply their brides with honey and at the marriage ceremony the groom promised to give his love twenty-four 'hins' of honey (about thirty-two pounds).

The Brahmans of Bengal anointed the bride's forehead, lips, eyelids and ear lobes with honey to ward off evil spirits and ensure a happy married life, and among some of the earlier Far Eastern races the bride would often be anointed with honey on her breasts and private regions to ensure fertility.

While for many honey has always been a source of food, and its pure nature increasingly endowed it with magical qualities, in some parts of the Middle and Far Eastern world it became endowed with aphrodisiac powers. Women, cattle and sometimes even food crops were expected to have greater fertility if honey figured in their religious ceremonies. In Morocco the Moors believed implicitly in honey as a love stimulant and large quantities of honey were used in their marriage ceremonies, which were more sex orgies than anything else, the bridegroom and guests consuming large quantities of honey, and wines and food made with honey.

An examination of many of the old recipes for love potions will show that basically they were made from honey. Although there is no medical or laboratory evidence to support the theory that honey has any aphrodisiac power at all, the late Dr Bodeg Beck, in his book *Honey and your Health*, probably provided the most likely explanation when he said:

> *Honey is rapidly assimilated and is an excellent source of quick energy. An anaemic, poorly nourished individual who was given an elixir made with honey would probably experience a sudden glow of well-being and renewed energy directly after taking it. There is nothing mysterious about this. Any half-starved creature who was given an easily assimilated food or beverage on an empty stomach would experience the same sensation. Otherwise, the power of honey as a love stimulant would depend wholly upon the individual's imagination.*

The Bible gives many references to honey both as a food and a sustainer of life.

Genesis gives us the first report of honey when Jacob sent Benjamin to Egypt with gifts of the 'best fruits of the land' which included balm, honey, spices and myrrh, nuts and almonds. And Palestine, the land settled by the Israelites after many years in the desert, is described many times as 'a land flowing with milk and honey'.

We are told by David's son Solomon, the wise one, 'Son, eat thou honey, because it is good, and the honey comb, which is sweet to thy taste.'

Again, to some people the story of Samson and his slaying of the lion with his bare hands is pretty commonplace. But some days later, when Samson again passed the place, he discovered that bees had taken up their abode in the carcass and from it he was able to gather some honey which he bore home to share with his mother and father. From this incident comes that well-known saying: 'Out of the strong came forth sweetness' which has led to disputes over the story's authenticity ever since. It is a fact that honey-bees will not remain near a stench or even strong odour, and therefore, say the sceptics, there is no truth in the story. However, it may be argued that in a country like Palestine where vultures would no doubt consume every vestige of flesh from the lion's carcass in a matter of hours, and the heat of the sun would whiten the bones, the rib cage of that lion could easily accommodate a swarm of bees, and the area abounds in wild honey-bee colonies.

Among the Palestinian tribes there are nomadic beekeepers, that is, beekeepers who move their bees from place to place in search of honey crops for their bees. Probably, their system of beekeeping derived from the days of the wandering tribes of Israel.

The ancient Greeks believed in the food value of honey. Many Greeks of the fifth century were dedicated to the furtherance of intellectual matters, the arts and a perfection of body and soul.

Among them were those who believed that honey would prolong life and endow the consumer with perpetual youth. Some made it an important part of their daily diet, believing that if they could get the correct food in the right proportions they could double their normal life-span. All Greek athletes were given honey as part of their diet and following any strenuous exercise or event a drink of honey and water very quickly banished fatigue. So noticeable was this that some thought it might be possible to eliminate tiredness altogether and in this way they would never grow old. Honey is used in much the same way by athletes today and is an important food ingredient of all the Olympic events that take place.

Pythagoras, the man who first broached the theory that the Earth was round, revolving in space, thought a great deal about prolonging life with a honey diet. He introduced bread and a generous amount of honey into his own diet and that of all his students, but one of the most popular diets among the Pythagorean School was said to be honey and milk. This later on became known as 'Ambrosia'.

Wholly liquid diets proved unsound in practice but the one chosen by Pythagoras, supplemented with fruit, nuts and vegetables, produced both a youthful appearance and sustained energy. The maestro himself lived to be ninety years old but one of his disciples, Appollonius, exceeded his master's age by twenty-three years.

Hippocrates, the Father of Medicine, advocated honey for long life and Democritus, the great physicist, who discovered the atom and said it was the basis of all matter, followed his brother intellectuals although he did experiment a great deal with his diet. However, apparently he found something that suited him because he lived to be 109, and at the end craved for death.

The legend goes that in his hundred-and-ninth year he decided to fast so that he might hasten his end, but the women of his household raised the very devil about it. They informed him that it was approaching the feast of Theomophoria, which was a three-day autumn feast for women, and it was most inconsiderate of him because if he died they would be denied the chance to attend under the customs of the time. In deference to their wishes he decided to remain alive until they returned from the festivities and he sipped hot honey, it is said, until it was more convenient for him to pass away.

In the days of the great Roman Empire honey was a familiar part of every Roman's diet and it figured in every feast and religious ceremonial.

The chronicles have it that towards the latter part of its influence and grandeur, Rome was given over to feasting, debauchery and depravity, especially during the period of Emperor Nero.

Most of us have heard of the Roman banquets at which the majority of those attending very often disported themselves in a manner unbecoming to normal human beings, and at which, it is said, violence and murder sometimes took place. On these occasions there would be many dishes in which honey was used. Both meats and poultry and game birds would be basted with honey and spices and cakes and sweets would also have honey as a main ingredient.

Whether the people ate too much or consumed too much wine is only a matter of conjecture, but the Romans certainly knew how to celebrate. Among the feasts were those covering the four seasons of the year, which would also be appropriate times to celebrate the honey harvests, and at which honey played an important part, for apart from honey being consumed the food and wine would also contain honey.

Beekeeping being a major industry of Rome it is natural that it would play an important part in any celebrations at the time, especially as large amounts of honey were exported to various parts of the empire.

There is no doubt at all that the Romans were great eaters—one might almost say, gluttons for food—but this went with the times and was not entirely confined to Rome. Wherever there was plenty- mostly as a result of conquest—there were those ready and willing to devour it, because one must understand that apart from a few items of food, such as honey, the seasonal products could not be stored for future use. Therefore the people rejoiced and celebrated at the appropriate time, when there was something with which to celebrate.

From the records of Pliny the Elder, who lived from A.D. 23 to his sudden death in A.D. 79, during the eruption of Vesuvius which overwhelmed Pompeii, we have come to learn a great deal of the medicinal and nutritional value of honey.

He believed that for good health and long life honey should be part of one's daily diet. He spent much of his time in travel through the then known world in search of material for his monumental *Natural History*. During the course of travel he visited Africa, Britain, Spain and many places around the Mediterranean and he was able to study the local records which often bore out his belief in honey.

In a survey of the northern areas of Italy he found that there were many people in the region between the River Po and the Appennines who were living to what one might term 'a ripe old age'. He also found that there was an association between them and the regular use of honey in their diet. Among these people were a number of bee-keepers and Pliny reports in his *Natural History* (seventh volume) that 124 of these individuals had passed their century, the oldest being 135 years old.

When he visited Britain Pliny wrote, 'These islanders consume great quantities of 'honey brew', meaning mead or mead ale. At the time of the Roman conquest. Britain was known as the Honey Isle of Beli, because a great deal of honey was produced throughout the British Isles. Apart from the large number of wild bee colonies living in the forests the Britons themselves would no doubt have been carrying on a crude form of beekeeping.

The earliest Christian centres in Britain encouraged beekeeping and it is through the monasteries that advances in beekeeping knowledge were made, for in the honey-bee abbots saw a good source of income and self-support. Indeed the produce of the hive provided food, light and drink in those far-off days. In fact, honey and bees-wax formed quite important commodities for many years, for in the Domesday Book there are records of the king's taxes being paid in honey and particularly beeswax. Under the then feudal system the lord of the manor would be responsible for the collection of produce from which he would extract the king's portion.

Reports of longevity among the people of the British Isles have been circulating for many years and church records, etc., have been cited showing that from time to time individuals have attained an extraordinary age before they died.

Unfortunately, the records of the times in which these people were born were not that reliable and so a score or more years could easily be added without any particular notice being taken. Indeed, it would not be difficult for an individual who had passed his four score years and ten to lose sight of his actual age and for some exaggeration to creep in. Particularly could this have happened in the case of Thomas Parr, a native of Shropshire, who died on 16th November 1635, said to have been 152 years old. He is said also to have married Catherine Milton at 102 and sired a son by her. It has been established that longevity was a trait of the Parr family and he led a rather quiet life, daily quaffing a good deal of mead, until he was invited to London, at the request of King Charles I, and there given a royal feast from which, it is said, he died. There might be some reasonable grounds for an error to have been made in the length of his life but he was still genuinely very old when he passed away.

Similar records to this have come out of Russia since the 1950s, where surveys similar to Pliny's have been carried out with equally astounding results. In the majority of cases these octogenarians have been found to be the local beekeepers, or to have some close association with beekeeping. In honour of one of these beekeepers, Eicarov Mamoud Baguir-Ogly, who attained the phenomenal age of 148 years, the Russians issued a commemoration postage stamp. But in addition to these people consuming daily doses of honey they have also been found to eat a great deal of the waste material that is left over after the honey is processed and strained. This would contain a large quantity of pollen and a certain amount of beeswax particles.

However overwhelming the evidence to show that where honey is used habitually longevity is the result, two further factors should be borne in mind. Firstly, among peasant folk and those poorly off, survival of the fittest would tend to be the rule, Nature ruthlessly weeding out the weak and establishing a strong constitution in the survivors, bestowing also agility, virility and a certain tenacity. Secondly, as beekeepers they would lead a quiet and generally sober life in tranquil surroundings which would add to their chances of a life longer than that of those engaged in far more vigorous pursuits. As a general rule beekeepers do live to a greater age than those occupied in other pursuits.

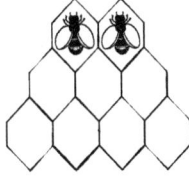

2
Honey in Legend and Mythology

As BEES were one of Man's earliest sources of food it is obvious that honey and the veneration of these insects have played a part in both his folklore and religious observances, almost from the beginning.

Although there is a great deal about bees and honey in Greek and Roman mythology, because both the Greeks and Romans practised beekeeping on a large scale, bees and honey play a significant part in all the major civilisations, and the record shows that the influence of the honey-bee stretched from the Far East to the westernmost tip of Europe. In fact it is believed by some that the cradle of the honey-bee was in India, and many references to bees are made in the *Rig-Veda*, one of the oldest sacred books of India, compiled some time between 2000 and 3000 B.C. Hilda Ransome, in her remarkable work *The Sacred Bee*, says that the *Rig-Veda* was written before the Aryans came to India. These Aryans spoke Sanscrit and through the Iranians of ancient Persia were probably connected in language and race with the principal European peoples. This may account for the resemblances in their literature and mythology.

Madhu is the Sanscrit word for honey which etymologically ties up with *methu* in Greek and Anglo-Saxon *medu*. Vishnu, Krishna and Indra were referred to as Madhava, meaning the nectar-born. Vishnu is represented by a blue bee on a lotus flower; Krishna, the incarnation of Vishnu, by a bee on his forehead.

About 1000 B.C. the caste system in India was in existence and the Laws of Manu, ancient writings of the time, state that no Brahman, highest of the four castes, may sell or trade in honey or wax and if he did so he was degraded to a lower caste of the agriculturalist.

If anyone stole honey, it was considered so valuable that in the next life, it was believed, he would be turned into a gad fly, and if a novice for the priesthood ate honey, which he might well do at the various feasts held in honour of their gods, he would have to fast three days and spend one day immersed in water.

When a male child is born in India honey is used in the birth-rite and while certain special formulae are recited the father of the child feeds the baby with honey, saying 'I give thee honey food so that the gods may protect thee and that thou mayest live a hundred autumns in this world.'

In marriage honey plays an important part in the religious ceremony and among Hindus today honey and curds are given to the bridegroom when he enters the bride's home. Honey is part of the ceremony and as the bridegroom kisses his bride he recites:

'Honey, this is honey, the speech of thy tongue is honey; in my mouth lives the honey of the bee, in my teeth lives peace.'

A swarm of bees going into a house in India portends bad luck; and to dream about bees settling on a house means ill will befall the house, as when a man dreams of bees entering his house he will die, or have great misfortune.

Among the Hittites, whose influence in Asia Minor was great from about 2800 to 700 B.C., beekeeping was quite advanced for they had laws and customs pertaining to the keeping of bees. There is little doubt that through them beekeeping and the European customs associated with bees and honey were transferred to people further east.

In Palestine, the land 'flowing with milk and honey', it is almost certain that beekeeping was a very well-established craft among the Hebrews long before the time of Christ. Many references to bees are made in the Talmud, and there are laws regulating the keeping of bees as well as references to honey in the Bible.

Because the Hebrew religion is herotheistic and Mohammedanism is monotheistic there are no mythological references to bees, but in the Koran one of the books is devoted to 'The Bee' and in it one reads:

> Thy Lord has taught the bee saying, provide thee houses in the mountains and in the trees, and in the hives that men do build for thee. Feed, moreover, on every kind of fruit, and walk the beaten paths of the Lord. From its belly cometh forth a fluid of varying hues, which yieldeth medicine for men. Verily in this is a sign for those who consider.

The bee is the only animal, says Mohammed, who is addressed by the Lord himself, and the 'fluid of varying hues' refers to the different colours of honey, and honey is good for healing as well as a food.

The following story illustrates this latter point:

A man went to Mohammed and said his brother had violent pains in his stomach, and the Prophet is said to have told him to give his brother honey. Later the man comes back and says his brother is no better. Mohammed says: 'Go back and give thy brother more honey, for God speaks the truth; thy brother's body lies.' When more honey is given the man recovers.

When Mohammed visited Paradise, according to the Sunna, a holy book, he found Christ who commanded the archangel Gabriel to give him three goblets, one of which was filled with honey. According to the Koran, rivers of honey flow in Paradise for the use of the god-fearing.

An Arab writer discoursing on Mohammed and his sayings wrote that the Prophet said:

> 'Honey is a remedy for every illness, and the Koran is a remedy for all illnesses of the mind, therefore I recommend you to both remedies, the Koran and honey.'

Greece, where there are more hives to the square mile than anywhere else in the world, and where the very famous Hymettus and Rose honeys originate, brings honey often into its literature and mythology.

Achilles is reported to have ordered oil and honey to be stood close to the funeral pyre of his friend Patrocles so that the food he so much enjoyed in life would be available in the nether world.

In Greece beekeeping has flourished from the days of antiquity, and even several hundred years B.C. there were honey and wax merchants. Honey has always been in great demand and in those far-off days the honey merchant supplied it to preserve the dead, especially if the person died in a foreign land and was being taken home for burial. Alexander the Great and Agesipolis, King of Sparta, were both anointed with honey to preserve their bodies.

One of the earliest myths wherein honey is mentioned, which is more widely known than some, concerns the birth of Zeus, whose father, Kronos, reigned over Olympus during the Golden Age, and whose fate had been foretold that he would be deposed by one of his sons. To make sure that this should not happen he took to swallowing each child his wife, Rhea, bore him. Five children were dealt with in this way until the birth of the sixth, Zeus. At this point Rhea drew the line, and to save the baby she had a stone wrapped in its clothes which Kronos, quite unsuspectingly, swallowed.

The infant was hidden in a cave on Mount Dicte in Crete where dwelt a colony of sacred bees who fed him honey, while a goat, Amaltheia, let him suckle her milk. The cave was guarded by armed men, the Kuretes, who, when the baby cried, covered his cries by clashing their armour and stamping their feet so that Kronos should not hear. The boy was reared successfully, later dethroned his father and became chief of the gods of Olympus.

The Muses, sometimes said to be the daughters of Zeus and Mnemosyne, conferred the gifts of sweet speech, poetry and eloquence upon men by sending bees to touch their lips. The young Pindar, while journeying to Thespiae, is said to have been overcome by the heat of the day and lay down to rest. While he was sleeping the bees came to his lips and covered them with honey, thus starting him off on his career of song which made him so renowned among the gods.

Lucan, Plato, Vergil and Sophocles are all said to have had their lips touched by honey whilst they were infants.

Theocritus writes of a goatherd, Comatas, who because he offered his master's goats to the Muses whom he served, was shut up in a cedar chest by the angry man. However, the bees came and fed him with honey, so that when at the end of the year the master opened the chest expecting to find Comatas dead, he found him alive and well.

The story of Glaucus, the son of Minos and Pasiphae, seems to confirm the supposition, often made, that the bee is a symbol of a new incarnation.

Hyginus, librarian of the Palatine Library, writing a version of the story, says:

Glaucus, while playing with his ball, fell into a jar of honey. His parents sought for him in vain and finally appealed to Apollo, who replied, 'A monstrosity has been born to you; whoso can detect the meaning shall restore your son to you.'

On hearing this oracle, Minos began to seek among his people for the monstrosity. He was told that a calf had been born, which three times a day, once every four hours, changed its colour, first being white, then red and lastly black.

To get the portent interpreted Minos called together his augurs, but they failed to find a solution until Polyidus, son of Keiranaus, compared the calf to the mulberry tree whose fruit is first white, then red, and finally turns black when fully ripe. Minos then told him, ' 'Tis thou who must restore my son.' Thereupon, Polyidus, while taking the auspices, saw an owl on a wine-bin frightening off some bees. He took this as an omen and removed the lifeless body of Glaucus from the jar.

Minos then told him that as he had found the body he must restore it to life, but he protested that this was an impossibility. But Minos was adamant and Polyidus found himself sealed in a tomb with the dead boy, and a sword in case he should fail. Shortly a snake appeared and glided towards the body. Polyidus, believing it to be after food, struck off its head with the sword. Then a second snake, coming in, search of the first, found it dead and returned for a certain herb with which it touched the body and restored it to life.

Polyidus uses the same technique on Glaucus, raises him from the dead and together they shout to attract attention. The boy's parents are delighted and Polyidus is rewarded by Minos with rich gifts.

Various versions of this story exist but it is the general supposition that the bees represented the soul trying to re-enter the dead boy who really did die and was buried in a jar of honey, and the owl prevented this.

Both in Germany and Scotland the belief existed that the souls of men departed their bodies in the form of bees, and this probably ties up with the ancient custom of 'telling the bees'. In Britain, as in many other parts of Europe, it was quite customary until recent times to 'tell' the bees whenever a person in the family died, particularly if it was the owner of the hives. Should this custom be neglected, it was considered, the bees would die.

The ritual attached to the 'telling' took a slightly different form from place to place, but as a rule the widow or family went to the hives, rapped three times, and said

'Bees, bees, thy master is dead,
Fly not away but remain to comfort me.'

Black crepe or ribbons were draped over the hives just before the funeral.

Some years ago an old beekeeper—well known among apiarists—died. On the day of his-funeral, as the coffin was carried down the path leading from his cottage followed by the family mourners, bees suddenly appeared as it were from nowhere, and followed the hearse to the church. Although the day was bright and sunny it was not particularly warm for bees; it was early spring. After the service in the little church, the coffin was brought out for burial, and there were the bees waiting to accompany the pall bearers to the graveside. No one was molested, and for some days after, the vicar says, the bees were to be seen around the grave.

Rather incredible, you may say, but the story was vouched for at the time by witnesses, who were themselves astounded.

Often the bee-soul came back to re-animate a body, so the ancients believed, and so it is not surprising that the following story should have arisen.

In the parish of Klein-Fetten, in Lower Engadine, some young men found an old woman lying prostrate on the ground as though dead. They carried her to a house nearby. Just as they laid her down a bee flew in through an open window, entering the gaping mouth of the woman who thereupon revived, and got up, and in a grumbling manner admonished her rescuers, telling them that next time anyone found her lying around they were not to touch her.

'Telling the bees' was not only confined to sad occasions such as death. All important events were conveyed to the hives because it was thought that only by this means could the beekeeper, or bee-master as he was called, ensure that his hives would be fruitful and supply him with much honey. In parts of southern Germany and Austria it was customary at weddings to dress the hives or the beehouse, a place where a lot of hives are kept together, with red cloth. In Dalmatia the bridegroom's mother presented the bride with a spoonful of honey, but as soon as the bride opened her lips to receive it the spoon would be withdrawn. This would be done several times before being suddenly pushed into her mouth.

When the bride entered the house this delightful little verse would also be sung by all present:

'The bride comes in a happy hour,
She has brought a blessing with her,
Round her head there gleams the sunlight.
In her hand there sits a falcon,
Peace and concord brings she with her,
In her mouth the honey's sweetness.'

The British Isles and Eire have a great tradition of legend and superstition surrounding honey-bees and honey.

In Lincolnshire it was believed that if a swarm of bees gathered on the dead bough of a living tree there would be a death in the beekeeper's family within twelve months; a similar belief existed in Wiltshire, while the country folk of Anglesey said that wheresoever on a tree a swarm alighted that part of the tree would die.

The Welsh are sure that good luck and prosperity follows wherever a strange swarm enters a garden or pitches on a house. If it enters the roof great prosperity will come to the owner of the house. In the north of England it is considered better to keep bees in partnership, then it is lucky, while in Northumberland sole ownership is never any good. To buy bees was certain to bring misfortune, for the bees would die. It was usual to trade a hive by barter.

Belief that bees in their hives make a loud buzzing sound or, as some said, sing a carol on Christmas Eve, was strong in many parts of Britain, particularly Gloucestershire and Monmouthshire, where it was the custom to form processions and visit the apiaries in the district to 'listen' to the bees. In the northern counties too the custom was followed and a certain Reverend Hugh Taylor writing about this quaint belief says: 'A man of the name of Murray died at the age of ninety, in the parish of Earsden, Northumberland. He told a sister of mine that on Christmas Eve the bees assembled to hum a Christmas hymn and that his mother had distinctly heard them do this on one occasion when she had gone to listen for her husband's return. Murray was a shrewd man, yet he seemed to believe this implicitly.' And many country folk were strongly of this belief even as recently as the beginning of this century.

It was also customary in other parts of Europe to visit the bees, notably in France, Germany and Switzerland. The performance was not quite the same, but in Switzerland certainly someone from the household had to listen to the hives at midnight on Christmas Eve.

Other festivities in France are also devoted to bees and honey. At Candlemas, for example, it is the proper thing to deck the hives with ribbons, and candles made from your own beeswax are blessed in the church. On Rogation Days the beekeeper must burn a candle to the Virgin Mary so that she will bless his bees to ensure good honey crops. In the Vosges beehives are decked with a consecrated crown on Corpus Christi Day, and on Good Friday palm crosses are fixed to the fronts of hives to bring prosperity for the year.

Swarming to the ancient beekeeper meant increase, honey and prosperity, but he looked to the bees to swarm early to obtain the best results, hence the jingle:

'A swarm of bees in May
Is worth a load of hay;
A swarm of bees in June,
Is worth a silver spoon;
But a swarm in July, Is not worth a fly.'

Down in Cornwall honey should be taken on St Bartholomew's Day (24th August) perhaps because he is reckoned to be the patron saint of bees, but there is some confusion on this point. Both Devon and Cornwall are agreed, however, that to move the beehives on Good Friday is lucky; any other time is likely to cause the death of the bees.

'Tanging' bees, or beating on an iron pot with a stick or key in order to get swarming bees to settle quickly, dates back to antiquity and was well-known among country folk up to the turn of the century. Its real purpose, rather than causing the absconding bees to settle on their owner's property, or return to the hive whence they came, was to indicate to others ownership. Under Roman law, which is woven into the pattern of most of our present laws, when bees leave their hive, as in a swarm, they are no longer the charge of the beekeeper but are classified as wild creatures— *ferae naturae*—and as such become the property of whoever can catch and hive them, unless the beekeeper, or his representative, can follow and keep them in sight until they settle. So when the beekeeper—or more often than not his wife—saw the bees rise in a great flying cloud, any vessel that lay handy and made a noise when banged vigorously was seized and pursuit of the swarm began.

On the Continent, and sometimes in Britain, the more devout beekeeper would cross himself as soon as he saw his bees swarm, then he would quickly gather up two handfuls of dry earth and throw it in the direction of the swirling bees. The fact that the bees often settled quickly, or even returned to their hive under this treatment, had very little to do with any religious invocation. The very simple explanation is that as the earth or fine dust begins to fall among the bees they immediately get the impression that it is raining and either settle close at hand, or rush back to the hive in order to avoid getting wet.

As weather prophets they are quite remarkable little creatures, for in the midst of a hot, sunny afternoon, when everything looks peaceful and calm, back will come the foragers from the fields, tumbling into their hives as though the Devil himself were after them, and slowly all activity in the apiary slows to a trickle. If this happens beware of rain; it won't be far away.

Or in the morning, when all the world looks grey and damp, look to the bees. When groups are seen flying hurriedly off to the fields, get out that picnic, leave your coat at home and go out to enjoy a fine, warm, sunny day, because it will be like that later on.

Bees can forecast the weather ahead too. Some days, or even weeks away from a prolonged spell of wet or cold conditions the bees make preparations. When drones and drone larvae are suddenly dragged from the hive and deposited outside be sure a bad spell of weather will follow one that looks set fair.

So much, much more could be written about the intriguing little creature we call the honey-bee; its social system quite unparalleled in the animal kingdom; its dance language of communication; its accuracy in indicating distance to its mates, and many other intricacies. But that would be deviating from the purpose of this book—to give the story, inadequate though it is, for we have much more to learn, of honey.

Much more could be written too of the superstitions and folklore surrounding the bee, but suffice it to give this final little story about the bee and the wasp:

At first God wanted to give the bee to the Romanians and the wasp to the gypsies.

God created the bee first because it is a creature that moves with the sun. However, the gypsies saw the bee and took it from God, saying that they needed it to provide food for themselves in the form of honey, and its beeswax they would use to light the church of God. God didn't say anything but meant to teach them a lesson. He therefore created the wasp, big and strong, which he offered to the Romanians, telling them that the bee had been ordained for the gypsies.

The Romanians took the wasp and thanked God most humbly.

In time the Romanians met the gypsies and the gypsies enquired how the Romanians were getting on with their wasps; had they collected much honey? Boastfully the Romanians replied that their wasps were big and strong and had filled many barrels with honey.

The wily gypsies thought to themselves, 'We must get those wasps', and when they were asked how they fared with the bees they answered that they had hardly filled a cup. 'But let us exchange our bees', they said.

Having agreed to do so the Romanians went with the gypsies and were given the bees which they took home. The gypsies then went with the Romanians to a forest where grew a very big tree, as wide as a barrel and reaching up into the heavens. There the Romanians had put the wasps, whose numbers had grown.

'Here you are', said the Romanians, 'Our bees are in this great hollow tree with honey enough to satisfy the whole gypsy nation.'

The Romanians went home to tend their new creatures, while the gypsies went to fetch a ladder and pots in which to put the honey. They climbed the ladder to where the wasps were flying but they were stung so unmercifully that they ran away; they'd had enough of wasps to last them for ever. The Romanians, of course, have kept bees ever since.

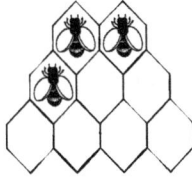

3
What is Honey?

FEW PEOPLE who eat honey ever stop to ask themselves this question. To most honey is a very nice sweet substance collected by bees and eaten by man for his sustenance and enjoyment. Few people even know that there are different kinds of honey which taste quite different from one another.

Honey is, however, a complex substance varying appreciably in its composition from flora to flora, country to country, soil to soil, and is even affected by climatic conditions. Thus a clover honey from Queensland, Australia, will show different characteristics from, say, clover honey from California, and both will differ in some respects from clover honey obtained in England. The main difference is in relation to the composition of the soil upon which the plant is feeding and more especially on the number of other plants growing in the same area at the same time and producing nectar. For example, an area predominant in clover blossom may have blackberry and lime blossom flowering and yielding nectar at the same time; whereas in another part of the world clover growing under similar conditions may have large quantities of lucerne in flower nearby, or sainfoin, or perhaps exotic plants such as one can find in Australia. All these minor honey sources can and do get mixed in a very natural way with the main bulk of clover honey as it is collected by each and every bee in the hive, yet because the main source is clover—probably 70 per cent—the honey will be known as clover honey.

Honey starts out as a very thin watery sugary fluid known as nectar. Nectar is found in the nectaries of plants which are usually located in the base of the flowers, although in some cases they may be found elsewhere; the laurel for instance secretes a similar fluid to nectar and offers it at the base of the underside of its leaves, especially young growth.

Nectar is the sweet offering of plants to honey-bees and other insects in return for the service these insects render in pollinating them. It's a case of providing food in return for a service.

Nectar varies considerably in its sugar and water content from one kind of a plant to another, as for example dandelion which has a nectar composed of approximately 60 per cent sugars and other components to 40 per cent water, whereas pear blossom has a water content as high as 70 per cent. The honey-bee is aware of this and goes for the higher sugar content whenever possible.

This dilute liquid is a solution of sucrose, or cane sugar, plus various other ingredients, and water. This is the substance the honey-bee extracts from the nectaries of each flower as she laboriously wings her way from floret to floret examining here, inspecting; there. In her quest for a single load of honey she may visit anything from 500 to 1,100 blossoms of a particular species of plant and, remember, a load represents only a small drop.

Inside the bee the nectar is stored in a tiny compartment known as the honey sac. This sac is like a little plastic bag fitted with a one-way valve, and here it undergoes its first change. For here are stored enzymes and juices which will convert the sucrose or cane sugar—commonly called a disaccharide—to more simple sugars known as monosaccharides. It is upon this conversion that nectar becomes known as honey, consisting mainly of two simple sugars, dextrose and levulose. The enzymes which play the main part in converting the nectar are invertase which brings about the change in the sucrose to dextrose and levulose; diastase which converts starch to the dextrines; catalose which decomposes hydrogen peroxide; and phosphatase which decomposes glycerophosphate.

This sounds all very complicated and it is, but to the honey-bee the whole process is a normal everyday occurrence during the warm flying days of summer, when she can get into the fields and woods among the myriads of sweet-smelling blossoms competing for her attention.

On the way back to the hive the nectar which the bee has collected is already undergoing its first change. For instance, in flight the bee will have absorbed a little of the water and the enzymes will have started their work of breaking down the sugars, and the dextrose and levulose will already be replacing the sucrose in the proportion of about 34 per cent of the former to 42 per cent of the latter. There are cases where the levulose exceeds 42 per cent and sometimes the dextrose is higher, but these will be described more fully later.

By the way, dextrose, or glucose as it is often described, and levulose or fructose are identical in chemical composition, but when viewed under the polarimeter, which is an instrument for measuring polarized light, the dextrose bends the plane of a ray of polarized light to the right while the levulose turns it to the left.

At the hive, or in the hollow of a tree, the worker bee either offers her load to a waiting worker, known as a house bee, and then skips off for another, or she may hurry to a cell in the combs and there deposit the droplet herself; it all depends how busy she is. If there is an intense honey flow on and flowers are yielding well the whole hive will be humming with activity. Then there will be no time for the foragers to do more than pass their collection on to the young house bees to store.

The 'unripe' honey as it is known at this stage has still a long way to go before it becomes 'ripe' and ready for sealing in the cell.

Firstly, a large proportion of the colony will evaporate off much of the water content of the honey. In this the bee uses quite a unique method of evaporation. It takes up a small quantity of the thin watery honey from a cell and then opening wide its mandibles, or jaws, it pushes its proboscis or tongue forward and downward. As a small droplet of thin liquid honey appears it is gradually extended until the whole is exposed as a thin film to the warm, dry currents of air in the hive, and in this way the honey rapidly loses its water content. When no more than 18 to 20 per cent of water remains the now ripened honey is sealed in a cell with a waxen cap where it is left to mature and finish its ripening process until claimed by the beekeeper or eaten by the colony as food.

If we were to take a sample of this honey and by means of special laboratory apparatus examine it minutely we would discover that it is quite a complex product consisting of the sugars, dextrose, levulose, sucrose and maltose; the acids cluconic, citric, malic, succinic, formic, butyric, lactic, pyroglutamic and amino; proteins, and an ash content containing the minerals potassium, sodium, calcium, magnesium, chlorides, sulphates, phosphates, silica, etc.

Further, we should find in minute quantity such substances as pigments, caratone, chlorophyll and chlorophyll derivatives and xanthophylls; flavouring which derives from terpens, aldehydes, alcohols and esters; sugar alcohols such as mannitol and dulcitol; tannins, inhibine which is a bactericidal substance very necessary, of course, to the honey in an atmosphere such as is found in the beehive; quite small quantities of vitamins such as thiamine, riboflavine, nicotinic acid, biotin, pyridoxine, and pantothenic acid, and as already mentioned, the enzymes.

This, then, will give you some idea of the complex substance which is honey, and to add to its complexity different honeys vary from one floral source to another. Add to this that there is still much to be learned about honey and its full composition and one soon begins to realise what a really intricate substance honey is and why it has intrigued and fired the imagination of man for thousands of years.

Both in the honey-bee and much more so in the cell of the hive, honey will also become mixed up with pollen which the bee collected as its protein diet, a substance which in itself is very highly complex in its composition and still not fully chemically explored. When honey is extracted out of the comb a large number of pollen grains of various plants will be present in it. Some of the larger size grains will later be filtered out in the filtering process which the beekeeper will give his honey, but very many remain as a highly nutritious ingredient of the honey.

At the present time something in the nature of fifteen different sugars have been identified in honey, although many of these sugars were not present in the original nectar but have come about during the ripening and maturing process in the hive, and are the result of enzymatic and acid action.

One of the outstanding physical properties of honey is its hygroscopicity—in other words its great natural attraction for moisture. This property makes honey very vulnerable to the normal moisture of the atmosphere. Should it become exposed to the air it soon takes up moisture to its detriment, for as the water content increases above 20 per cent so the yeasts which most natural products possess become active and lead to fermentation unless their activity is checked in time.

The hygroscopicity of honey, on the other hand, gives honey a great natural healing power, for disease germs cannot thrive in its presence and are rapidly destroyed as it -denies them water in which to live. But more of this later on when we come to discuss the great healing properties of honey. This property will also be discussed in relation to the use of honey in cake-making.

Minerals in honey have already been mentioned and their presence varies widely from one honey to another, the darker honeys generally containing the larger amounts although, like the vitamin content, they are pretty small.

Today we all know how important it is to maintain the mineral content of our bodies for when the body becomes bereft of part of its minerals there is loss of energy and vitality. In severe cases of mineral deficiency lassitude of mind and body develops. Honey does not contain any great quantity of minerals as compared with some other food products, but added to any normal diet it must increase the mineral intake, and in this respect alone honey cannot be compared to any of the artificially produced sugars.

If we look at the mineral requirements of our body we find that calcium and phosphorus top the list whilst potassium, chlorine, sulphur, sodium and magnesium follow closely on. Other minerals needed for bodily health but in such small requirements as to be known as trace elements are copper, iodine, iron manganese, zinc, molybdenum and fluorine.

Iron is extremely important to the bloodstream, being a constituent of haemoglobin and also several enzymes which are necessary in oxidative reactions. Manganese is most important to many enzyme systems and is the primary metal for the enzymes of the citric acid cycle, the scheme of metabolism wherein most of the final oxidation to carbon dioxide occurs.

Dark honeys are usually richer in minerals than the lighter ones as will be seen from the opposite, which table is taken from *The Hive and the Honey Bee* and rearranged from Schuette *et al.*

It is difficult to say what importance the vitamin content of honey has for us because the quantity of vitamins is so small. However, they can be measured and they vary in assay from one honey to another. Their presence in honey is ascribed to the pollen content, and the more pollen present the higher the value of vitamins.

With a new and more highly developed technique for determining the vitamin content of food more light has been shed on these important constituents of our daily nourishment.

Professor M. H. Haydak at the University Farm, St Paul, Minnesota, U.S.A., with a group of research workers, undertook a study of a number of American honeys some years ago and he came up with some interesting data on the subject. Other researchers, notably Kitzes, Schuette and Elvekjem, have also added to our knowledge of the vitamins in honey, but it is a fact that with highly efficient filtering equipment there is a notable loss of vitamins, as also when heat is applied in processing honey.

An interesting and important find has been that honey is an excellent medium for vitamin stability whereas fruits and vegetables lose a considerable proportion of their vitamin content on storage.

Mineral Constituents of Honey
(parts per million)*

Element	Number of samples†	Light Honeys			Dark Honeys		
		Average	Mini-mum	Maxi-mum	Average	Mini-mum	Maxi-mum
Potassium	13, 18	205	100	588	1676	115	4733
Chlorine	10, 13	52	23	75	113	48	201
Sulphur	10, 13	58	36	108	100	56	126
Calcium	14, 21	49	23	68	51	5	2
Sodium	13, 18	18	6	35	76	9	400
Phosphorus	14, 21	35	23	50	47	27	58
Magnesium	14, 21	19	11	56	35	7	126
Silica (SiO_2)	14, 21	22	14	36	36	13	72
Silicon (Si)	10, 10	8.9	7.2	11.7	14	5.4	28.3
Iron	10, 10	2.4	1.2	4.8	9.4	0.7	33.5
Manganese	10, 10	0.30	0.17	0.44	4.09	0.52	9.53
Copper	10, 10	0.29	0.14	0.70	0.56	0.35	1.04

* The parts per million equal the milligrams per kilogram, or divided by 10,000 equal the actual per cent of the total honey composition.

† The first figure refers to the number of samples of light honeys, while the second figure refers to the number of samples of dark honeys.

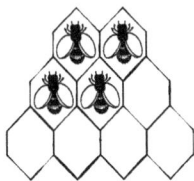

4

Honeys of the World

LARGE SECTIONS of the population of honey-consuming countries only recognise honey under a particular brand name, thus up to the Second World War and since, the vast majority of honey offered for sale in grocers shops in Britain has been a blend of various honeys obtained usually from Australia, Jamaica, the Middle East or the American continent. One or two well-known packers, famous thirty or more years ago, handled either Australian, New Zealand or Canadian clover honeys, and these topped the sales of honey in this country. Similar conditions applied to the sale of honey in the United States where the bulk of. the product was home-produced but mostly sold as a blended product under various trade marks.

When the Second World War got under way food rationing followed and with it a curtailment of honey imports and indeed every kind of sweet, including sugar.

The rationing of sugar drove hundreds of people to find a means of securing their own sweets; they became beekeepers and by the end of hostilities every country where honey-bees could be kept had greatly expanded its beekeeping, far out of proportion to its pre-war status. During this period the normal offering of honey by the grocers had materially dwindled but a thriving local industry in honey sprang up and it was usually only procurable from the producer. But something else also happened. With the new type of honey, people began to get an appetite for special honeys. True, the majority of home-grown honey was offered under a label proclaiming it to be 'English' honey, but one honey tasted different from another. There were clover, hawthorn, lime, blackberry and heather honeys, in fact, honeys to match the major sources of flora available to the honey-bees; and the public learned to appreciate the subtle differences in sweetness and bouquet of these honeys.

After the war, rationing persisted for a period, and countries like America, Canada and Britain continued to expand their national beekeeping activities. Honey was being sold at a very high premium despite government control and legislation. People wanted honey and were prepared to pay for it.

When rationing ended and normal trading was restored large quantities of foreign honeys began to filter into the economies of various countries which had previously been large importers, Germany being one of the largest. The restoration of sugar supplies also made a difference; honey sales for a very short while took a dip and the local beekeeper found himself carrying stocks. This was a new experience and by 1950 there was an extraordinary amount of surplus stocks of honey everywhere, not only in Britain but in most other honey-producing countries.

Australia had bumper harvests of honey around the years 1947 to 1949, and she was forced to unload on to countries like Germany and Britain. Prices were forced down but the old range of honey coverage was restored and the housewife once again had a choice of a cheap foreign, or expensive local, honey. Everything looked set for honey trading to return to the position it had held before the war, but the packers had not reckoned with the changing conditions which had been brought about by the war itself. Honey farming in countries like Australia and America had greatly increased to meet the public demand. Two brilliant Germans interned in Mexico at the outbreak of the war decided to stay on and develop the largest and most prosperous beekeeping business in the world. In fact the success of their venture is almost like a fairytale. The Miel Carlotta honey company, as it is known, is never quite sure of the actual number of colonies of bees it really does own, although it was last estimated at 68,000. And all this started from two hives of bees and the determination of two individuals to kill boredom. Their influence also provoked other Mexican honey producers to expand and modernise their honey plants. In South America beekeeping took on a new significance and Argentina has topped the list of exporting countries during the last ten years, exporting as much as 30,000 tons in a year.

While New Zealand has fallen behind with her honey production she still exports fairly large quantities of honey but nothing like the volume that she did before the Second World War. Her place is now being taken by China, although the quality of Chinese honey varies enormously despite the fact that all honey is channelled. through state-controlled honey plants.

Europe too has expanded her honey production since the war and countries like Poland, Spain, Hungary, Romania, Greece and France do regular but relatively small business with honey-importing countries.

The result of these new and quite exciting offers of honey, generally of uniflora origin, was the start in Britain of a new trend in honey. Although several companies had begun it before 1939 on a quite small scale, one firm sprung into existence offering a wide range of honeys based on country of origin and floral designation. Others followed. Thus one could buy, say, Spanish Orange-Blossom honey, Rosemary honey, Californian Sage honey, or Australian Clover, or Yellow Box and many others. All deliciously appetising, and novel taste experiences.

The trend widened and grew, and with it the honey consumption of the world began to expand as never before. Today it looks large by comparison with yesterday, but the desire for honey as one of nature's most natural, unadulterated sweets is as yet only scratching the surface; by tomorrow, today's consumption will look infinitesimal by comparison, for the health benefit of honey is only just beginning to be rediscovered since it fell into disuse with the advent of sugar.

For a better appreciation of the world's uniflora honeys it is best to examine them country by country.

Australia, land of sunshine and exotic and unusual flora, is today perhaps the world's largest honey producer, but by tomorrow it will be an even greater potential source of honey. Due to the intense sunshine, high temperatures and dry conditions plants store nectar in copious quantities, particularly the trees which give long and heavy honey flows from their myriads of blossoms. Unfortunately, some trees like the eucalyptus produce a honey with a strong, pungent taste and odour, which although often appreciated by the local inhabitants is not acceptable to the rest of the world. This is why years ago Australian honey got a name for poor quality, whereas it is a country, like every other honey-producing country, that has high quality, medium quality, and quite poor honeys. The latter are only fit for manufacturing purposes, and every year large quantities of this low-grade honey go into a wide variety of products such as tobacco curing, cough mixtures, breakfast cereal manufacture and even some beauty preparations.

From Australia we get such honeys as *Yellow Box* from the plant of that name. This is a very mild, light yellowy honey which, because of its high levulose sugar content, takes many months to granulate. It is an ideal honey for use on breakfast cereals, for sweetening fruit drinks or for use in cakes which have a delicate taste.

Blue Gum and *Red Gum*, on the other hand, are somewhat stronger in flavour and darker in colour. Both have a very pleasant flavour and bouquet, Red Gum reminding one very much in taste of raisins.

Australia, like most honey-producing countries, has also its *Clover* honey, and the best examples come from Queensland. This is a honey that is much sought after by the local people and Clover-honey eaters all over the world.

One would hardly associate *Mugga Mugga* with the name of a honey but it is a most delightfully flavoured honey which granulates or candies with a smooth fine grain. *Iron Bark* may conjure up strange thoughts but the tree of this name produces a honey which is both delightful and as fragrant as its blossom.

Tasmania, Australia's near neighbour, is best known for its *Leatherwood* honey which some claim is one of the most delightful in the world. In colour the honey is a light amber but the slightly scented bouquet and taste leaves a lingering desire for more.

The Leatherwood tree is mostly found in the southern part of the island where beekeepers move hundreds of hives in the spring to await the opening of the first small white blossoms which give off a most fragrant scent, attracting the thousands of bees in the neighbourhood. About two years ago, following severe drought conditions, huge fires broke out and swept the area, destroying hundreds of acres of the Leatherwood trees and about a third of the honey bees, resulting in a temporary shortage of the honey.

From New Zealand has come for very many years a very fine pale amber-coloured *Clover* honey. This honey has found favour in England and in those countries where the population has a palate for the sweet and milder honeys.

In marked contrast to this there is a dark, rather pungent honey from the same country, *Manuka*, from the plant of that name. Unlike pretty well every other kind of honey, but very much akin to English or Scottish Heather honey (*Calluna vulgaris*), Manuka has a jelly-like consistency. In fact after it has stood a while it reminds one of jelly but as soon as it is agitated it runs naturally like ordinary honey. This is known as thixotropy and the reason for this peculiar nature is the presence in the honey of a protein not unlike the white of an egg. The Germans are very fond of Manuka honey and large quantities are imported every year.

In the United States of America, like Australia, there is a quite remarkable range of honeys which are being exploited a little more as uniflora honeys than they were twenty years ago. Some are remarkably smooth and rich-tasting with quite the most interesting bouquets. Like Tasmanian Leatherwood the bouquet lingers long after.

Honeys range in colour from water white, of which a good example is *Willowherb* (or Fireweed, because it grows where fires have been; the bomb sites of London were full of this plant after the last war), to dark amber such as *Buckwheat* gathered in large quantities around New York State, Ohio and Michigan. It is also part of the honey crop of Canada. More than sixty kinds of pure source honey have been identified in the U.S.A., but again the finest of honeys are the clover honeys of Montana, Minnesota and the Middle West states generally.

However, for distinctive tasting honey California is foremost with its light amber *Orange Blossom*, a honey of thick density. Sage is somewhat darker in colour but with quite an unusual flavour, a property shared by honeys with such high-sounding names as *Star Thistle, Sourwood, Mesquite* and *Mountain Thyme*.

Grapefruit honey of Texas is said to be a connoisseur's choice, but *Tupelo* from the swamps of Florida could also rank in this category too. This latter honey has a distinction of remaining in liquid form because of its high levulose sugar content.

Alfalfa, sweet clover and alsike clover are not only valuable forage crops for animals but also contribute a valuable proportion of the honey collected in the northern states. The United States is said to have more than 1,800 different trees, shrubs and plants from which honey-bees collect nectar, and there are something in the region of fifty agricultural crops which are dependent on bees for pollination and these, of course, produce small or large quantities of nectar depending upon the acreage under cultivation.

In America the use of insecticides has greatly reduced the number of wild pollinating insects as well as honeybees, so that there is a great demand for hives of bees, and beekeepers move their bees about from apple to apricot, almond to avocado. Every year the vast orchards of this great country hire trailer loads of bees just to secure a good fruit set, and the tremendous acreages of alfalfa and other seed crops command the services of beekeepers and their bees as well.

Some large beekeeping outfits, where there may be anything from 3,000 to 10,000 hives, move up and down the country from north to south and back again according to the season. These migratory beekeepers follow the sun and the crops of honey with their equipment set up on caravans; home and all. Even the extracting of honey is dealt with on the spot. Among the largest operators are those who have their own aeroplanes for location spotting and whose owners prospect in advance of a move in order to obtain the most advantageous sites, promising the best honey flows.

Mexico has rapidly developed as a honey-producing country since the war and is one of the leading exporters. In a good year her beekeepers can offer as much as 25,000 to 30,000 tons of quite good grade honey. Much of the surplus honey comes from the Yucatan and Campeche areas. Yucatan honey is generally a blend of main crop honeys which the bees have usually collected over a very wide area of flora from some of the tiniest plants to the forest trees. However, there are uniflora honeys like *spring apple blossom* and *guadalajara*, two light amber honeys of excellent flavour.

Because Mexican honey is both cheap and carries a good flavour it is much in demand in Europe and every year its popularity increases.

Honeys procured from the forest flowers of Guatemala and that which comes from Jamaica are all honeys that are reasonably cheap because they are collected and packed in a rather rudimentary fashion, but for all that they are honeys of good flavour and high food value and once the packers take them in hand they can be carefully filtered and processed to a very high standard.

It is claimed by some that because these honeys are collected by the bees in relatively primitive conditions where there is a noted absence of insecticides and other agricultural chemicals, there is no possible contamination and therefore from a health-food point of view they are more desirable, but this is debatable.

Europe generally is a continent where a variety of superior honeys are harvested by the bees for distribution to many places. France, for example, can boast of some of the most delectable honeys, *Rosemary* from the Narbonne and Languedoc districts, *Heather* honey, both *Erica* and *Calluna*, from the areas about the south-west, *Lavender* from the Pyrenees, *Jasmine*, *Acacia* and *Sycamore*, the latter having a greenish tinge but prized as a honey speciality.

The finest Acacia (*Robinia suedo-acacia*) honey comes from Hungary, Romania and Yugoslavia. In 1954 I was in Serbia during May and June and there I saw the bees gathering the honey from the massed blossom of the acacia trees that lined the banks of the river Sava, and it appeared to be pouring into the great 'coffin' hives, so fast was the traffic in bees. Acacia honey is a quite pale yellow colour, rather insipid to some palates but very viscous, remaining liquid for an extraordinarily long time on account of its high levulose content.

It was while staying in Yugoslavia that I discovered honey shops where the principal commodity was honey, and folks just came along with their jugs or jars and purchased honey loose from great vats, much as one bought milk in England before the food laws forbade it.

Spain produces some interesting honeys but their chief export is *Orange Blossom* and *Rosemary*, and tourists are offered *Lavender* honey.

Germany, like England, is a bigger importer of honey than a producer, but there is a relatively large number of hobbyist beekeepers who produce a wide variety of honeys. Their most prized and most expensive product comes from the pine forests and is really a honey-dew (the saccharide exudation of the aphids that feed from the pine needles). It is dark brownish in colour with an accompanying strong taste and is considered a great delicacy and much relished. From the Luneberg Heath district of Germany, depending upon the weather, comes a quite good Heather honey.

And *Heather* honey reminds me that the finest of this type of honey derives, without a doubt, from Scotland and the northern counties of England. Heather (*Calluna vulgaris*) is obtained in other districts, from a number of counties in the south, and from Wales, but I never think it compares to the full with that produced by the bees on the heather moors, fells and highlands of the north.

Lime honey is to be found in most countries, but for some reason or other—and one can only think it must be soil—Poland produces a perfectly good Lime honey which carries a slight greenish tinge but the most pleasant of flavours.

Another tree honey which finds favour with the honey connoisseur is *Sycamore*, but to look at it the uninitiated might think it rather dull because it has that appearance. When first gathered, too, it sometimes has a 'green' taste but after a couple of months this disappears and is replaced by an extremely pleasant mellow flavour.

In the north of England, where very often a large spring crop of Sycamore honey is gathered, usually mixed with a generous proportion of other spring flowers such as hawthorn, there is a premium on its sale. Hawthorn itself is a spasmodic yielder and only about once in five years do the bees collect surplus honey from this most beautiful of England's hedgerow and woodland plants. When they do the beekeeper shakes his head for the rest of the season very, very often proves a disaster.

F. N. Howes, in his book *Plants and Beekeeping*, lists the following as the major sources of honey in the British Isles. They are: Clover, Lime, Heather (both *Calluna vulgaris* and *Erica cinerea*). Fruit Blossom, Sainfoin, Mustard and Charlock, Hawthorn, Sycamore, Blackberry, Willowherb, Field Beans, Buckwheat and Dandelion.

Of the above list it is doubtful if charlock, sainfoin and buckwheat can be called major honey plants of England, for charlock has been largely eliminated by chemical sprays and the other two are never grown on the same scale as before the Second World War.

And it would be quite out of place to close this chapter without reference to two world-famous honeys —Greek *Hymettus* and Greek *Lemon Blossom*; both carry the mark of quality and the fragrance of Nature.

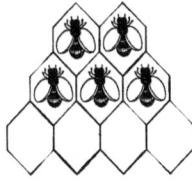

5

Food of the Gods

WITH THE greatly increased demand for honey of all kinds these days there must inevitably follow a demand for cookery ideas and recipes in which honey can be incorporated, especially as more and more is learnt of the wide range of flavours associated with honeys from different plants and countries.

Although it is not always realised, honeys differ from one another as delicate wines do and it can be said with truth that there are good and average vintage years for honey just as there are vintage years for wines. In fact good wine years and honey years generally coincide, in as much as it takes hot sunny summers to produce both.

Those who like honey are not always aware that it has far more uses than for just spreading on bread and butter, or maybe for easing for coughs and colds.

Unfortunately honey is not the easiest of materials to handle as it is sticky and difficult to pour readily from most containers. This is probably the reason why women generally turn to such sweetening agents as granulated sugar or the more pourable commercial syrups. Furthermore, without a little enlightenment honey can present a problem when used to replace sugar completely in cooking, especially cake-making. Few people realise that honey contains 18 to 20 per cent water and therefore this should be allowed for in any recipe. If then the cook calculates for one-fifth less liquid for any liquid that is to be added, and if the recipe calls for, say, 10 ounces of sugar, she realises that 12 ounces of honey is the required replacement, there should be little difficulty with the result.

Honey runs more readily when warm, so if you want to avoid a heavy unmanageable stream when pouring it, warm it up first. Better still, take a small quantity from the main container and put it into a small jug with a good clean-cut spout.

For occasions when honey is required for sweetening cereals or porridge mix a little hot water with a small quantity. In this way it will pour perfectly and cover the cornflakes or porridge with a fine spreadable stream, but when it is used in this manner see that it is used up almost at once otherwise any left over will have the tendency to ferment.

A disappointment to many honey consumers is when they find that they are only half-way through a jar of honey and it begins to go cloudy and then from a bright liquid it turns sugary and sometimes even takes on a set solid condition.

All pure honey, with a few exceptions, like Acacia, Tupelo, etc., crystallises or granulates, and unless it has had prolonged heat treatment at temperatures which can harm its structure, liquid honey regranulates after a comparatively short time, specially in temperatures below 60° F or 15 °C. Therefore it is quite obvious that a jar of honey will start to regranulate if left for a period but this is by no means detrimental to the honey. If it is placed in a pan of hot water and left for a while it will again become liquid. In more stubborn cases it might be necessary to put a little heat under the pan to completely reconstitute it, but that is all.

It might not be out of place here to mention something about the use of honey as regards flavour.

If you are thinking of substituting honey for, say, artificial sugar in tea, choose a mild honey like Clover or Acacia. They are sweet but not strong-tasting. Honeys with a more distinct flavour can be used in coffee or stronger-flavoured fruit drinks where the flavour of the honey is masked by the flavour of the beverage, but remember there are a few honeys that have such strong tastes that they should never be used in the culinary arts at all. For example, Australian dark amber, New Zealand Manuka, or any Heather honeys.

Some discernment should be used when baking cakes with honey. A madeira should have only a light honey such as Clover, Alfalfa, or Acacia, whereas it would be quite permissible to put Hawthorn or Mexican Yucatan in a heavy fruit cake, thereby improving its general flavour.

The important value of honey in cake-making or bread-making is its moisture-retaining property and cakes made with honey keep far longer than those made with sugar.

Toasted bread, scones or flapjacks are delicious with a generous helping of, say, Orange Blossom honey or Mexican Yucatan. This is where a cut-off drizzle jug such as is used on the Continent and in America is very handy, because a measured amount of honey can be delivered on to the article without drippy stickiness resulting.

During the past twenty-five years a number of excellent honey cookery recipe books have been published, prompted no doubt by the wide publicity given to honey and honey cookery by such organisations as the American Honey Institute of Madison, Wisconsin, and the Australian Food and Wine Bureau. Most of the very ancient dishes which have been rediscovered are probably the result of the constant research that is going on into the past history of cookery all over the world.

It would be quite impossible within the scope of this book to offer all the mouth-watering and scrumptious honey recipes that are available. If the reader desires to go further there are specific works on this subject alone and, of course, several good centres continually experimenting with new recipes, but here are some from a long list which I have collected during the past thirty years and used with great satisfaction.

Honey Bread and Cakes

Although honey can replace sugar in almost all cookery recipes, when it comes to cake-making the experts argue that a certain amount of sugar is necessary to guarantee that the article will turn out perfect and not too moist or even underdone. And to those who have 'a thing' about eating white sugar, there is little doubt that in cake-making its unhealthy nature is greatly diluted or lost in the rest of the ingredients.

Ginger Honey Cake
3 ozs. butter   2 ozs. light brown sugar   1 egg and 1 egg yolk
6 ozs. wholemeal self-raising flour   pinch of salt   1 dessertspoon ground
ginger   1 teaspoon cinnamon   2 tablespoons honey   6 tablespoons milk

Pre-heat oven to moderate (gas 350°, electric 375°). Grease a 7" round tin with butter and line the bottom with paper. Cream butter, sugar and honey together. Beat in 1 egg plus 1 yolk. Mix in sifted ingredients alternately with the milk. Turn into prepared tin and bake 40-45 minutes. Yields 24 slices.

Australian Honey Board

Coconut Cookies
2ozs. desiccated coconut   2ozs. plain flour pinch of salt   1 oz. sugar
2 ozs. butter or margarine   1 tablespoon honey   glacé cherries

Sieve flour and salt into basin. Add coconut. Rub in butter. Add sugar and honey and knead mixture well until it clings together in one large ball. Flour the hands and roll mixture into small balls. Put on to greased baking sheets and flatten with the thumb. Place a small piece of cherry on each.. Bake in a moderate oven for 15 to 20 minutes.

Honey Cookery—Ambrose Heath

Honey Fruit Cake
1 cup honey   ½ lb. butter   5 eggs   1 cup dates   2½ cups plain flour
2 teaspoons baking powder   4 tablespoons allspice   2 cups chopped raw
peanuts   1 cup chopped almonds   2 cups currants   2 cups seedless raisins
¼lb. mixed peel   ¼ lb. crystallised pineapple   ½lb. candied cherries

Sift flour, measure and divide into two equal parts. To one add baking powder and all-spice, and sift twice more. Cream butter well. Add honey. Add well-beaten egg yolks. Add sifted dry ingredients gradually. Fold in stiffly-beaten egg whites. Roll nuts and fruits (except cherries and pineapple) in remaining flour. Add to the dough mixture. Add cherries and pineapple. Bake in 9" tin in slow oven 2½ hours or more.

Australian Honey Board

Honey Tea Cakes
1 lb. flour   2 tablespoons melted butter   pinch of salt   2 large tablespoons
baking powder   2 tablespoons honey   2 eggs   a little milk

Beat the eggs thoroughly and add the other ingredients with sufficient milk to make a light dough. Drop with a spoon into greased patty tins and bake for 10-15 minutes at 425° gas, 450° electric.

Australian Honey Board

Applesauce Cake
⅓ cup shortening ¾ cup honey 2 cups flour ¼ teaspoon cloves
½ teaspoon cinnamon ½ teaspoon nutmeg ¼ teaspoon salt
1 teaspoon bicarbonate of soda 1 cup cold applesauce (unsweetened)
1 cup seedless raisins.

Cream shortening. Add honey gradually, creaming after each addition. Mix and sift together dry ingredients and add alternately with the applesauce to the creamed mixture. Fold in raisins. Pour batter into a well-greased 8" x 8" pan. Bake in a moderate oven (350° F) for about 45 minutes.

American Honey Institute

Honey Meringue
1 egg white ½ cup honey

Beat egg white with rotary or electric beater until it begins to froth. Then add honey, gradually beating until meringue stands high in peaks (from 5 to 10 minutes beating). Use on puddings or cakes.

Where a hand rotary is used it is recommended that the honey is warmed through gently for 10 minutes, left to cool slightly, then the egg whites added and the mixture beaten.

American Honey Institute

Nurnberg Pastries
5 ozs. honey 2 eggs 1½ ozs. halved almonds 1 oz. grated orange peel 1 oz. chopped candied peel crushed cloves cinnamon 5 ozs. flour

Beat up the honey with the eggs until well blended. Stir in the halved almonds, grated orange peel, chopped candied peel, crushed cloves, cinnamon, and the flour. Roll out the pastry very thinly and place on a well-greased baking tray. Cook in a moderate oven. Cut the pastry into strips and return to the oven for a short time to dry before cooling.

Honey Cookery—Stadtlaender

Honey Sponge
3 eggs ¾ cup honey 1 teacup (4 ozs.) self-raising flour pinch of salt
2 dessertspoons cold water

Beat whites of 2 eggs with honey until stiff. Beat yolks with remaining egg. Gently stir into first mixture. Fold in flour sifted with salt, and lightly mix in water. Bake in well-greased sandwich tins in moderate oven. Suggested filling: 2 tablespoons butter, 2 tablespoons honey, few drops vanilla essence. Beat to a soft cream.

Australian Honey Board

Honey Fruit Loaf
>   3 oz. butter   3 ozs. light brown sugar   2 tablespoons honey   1 egg
>   8 ozs. self-raising wholemeal flour   ¼ teaspoon salt 1 teaspoon mixed spice
>   1 cup mixed fruit, cut small   4 tablespoons milk

Pre-heat oven to moderately hot (gas 375°, electric 400°). Grease an oblong loaf tin 9" x 3" x 3" with butter. Cream butter and brown sugar. Add egg and honey, then wholemeal flour, salt and spice alternately with the milk and fruit. Place in prepared tin and bake for 40-45 minutes. Yields 24 half slices.

>   Australian Honey Board

Yuletide Flapjacks
>   6 ozs. plain flour 2 eggs ½ pint milk 1 oz. butter   4 tablespoons honey
>   2 tablespoons brandy   caster sugar   pinch of salt

Sieve the flour and salt into a basin and make a well in the centre. Break in the eggs and gradually incorporate the flour, using a wooden spoon. Add half the milk, gradually, and beat the mixture until smooth. Now add the remaining milk. Cover the mixture and allow it to stand for 30 minutes. Heat a small piece of the butter in a frying-pan and pour in sufficient of the batter to make a thin layer on the bottom of the pan. Cook until a golden brown on one side, then turn by tossing in the traditional manner; cook until golden brown on the other side. Mix the honey and brandy together and spread on the flapjacks while they are still hot. Roll up, sprinkle with caster sugar and serve. This recipe should produce 12 flapjacks.

Honey Tea Cakes
This is a useful item at teatime when you may have run out of other ideas.
>   2 breakfast cups fine white flour   level teaspoon baking powder
>   ½ level teaspoon bicarbonate of soda ½ level teaspoon salt 2 eggs
>   ½ breakfast cup clear honey 1 level teaspoon lemon essence
>   1 breakfast cup thick sour cream   lemon icing (optional)

Sieve together the flour, baking powder, bicarbonate of soda and salt. Beat the eggs until they become frothy; gradually beat into them the clear honey and lemon essence. Now add the flour mixture alternately with the sour cream, beating the mixture after each addition to smoothness. Turn into small greased muffin tins and bake in a moderate oven for about 20 minutes. Can be eaten as they are, or iced with a lemon icing.

Honey Snaps
>   2ozs. margarine 2ozs. sugar 2ozs. plain flour
>   1 level teaspoon ground ginger   2 tablespoons honey

Melt the margarine, sugar and honey together in a saucepan. Add the flour and ginger sieved and mix together. Drop teaspoonsful on to a well-greased baking tray (2 or 3 per tray to allow for spreading). Bake in a moderate oven for 7 minutes until golden brown. Allow to cool on the tray for 2 minutes before rolling round the handle of a wooden spoon. When cold they can be filled with cream before eating. Quite delicious!

Honey Buns

4 ozs. medium or light-coloured honey (Acacia, Clover or Australian light amber) 2 eggs 4 ozs. self-raising flour glace cherries

Gradually beat the egg yolks into the honey, add the flour and the stiffly-whisked whites of the eggs. Add a few chopped up glace cherries. Put dessert spoonsful of the mixture into buttered patty tins, with a glace cherry in the centre of each. Bake in a moderate oven until golden brown.

Honey and Nut Gateau

½ lb. honey 6 eggs 2 ozs. plain flour 2½ ozs. nuts pounded with a little sugar cream to bind

Melt honey carefully over hot water, beat the egg yolks in a bowl, and pour the honey over them. Now add slowly the flour and nuts. Then pour in enough cream to bind the mixture, and lastly fold in the beaten egg whites. Bake in a moderate oven in a buttered souffle dish or cake tin for approximately 40 minutes. Turn out when cold.

Fried Pastries

2 ozs. sultanas 8 ozs. plain flour 4 ozs. margarine ½ teaspoon baking powder pinch of salt a little water shallow fat for frying

Sieve the flour into a basin, add salt and baking powder, rub in the margarine, add sultanas and mix with sufficient cold water to make a stiff dough. Roll out to about a ¼ inch thick, cut into rounds and fry immediately in hot fat. Serve very hot, split, spread with a medium or light honey and put together like sandwiches.

No layer cakes or sandwich sponges are complete without their fillings and the success of these cakes depends upon that final touch. Two such fillings that come readily to mind are given in *Old Favourite Honey Recipes*, issued by the American Honey Institute.

Lemon Honey Filling

¼ cup sugar 2 tablespoons flour ¼ cup lemon juice ½ cup honey grated rind of 1 lemon 1 egg, lightly beaten 1 tablespoon butter

Mix ingredients in top of a double saucepan. Cook over hot water, stirring constantly until thickened. Cool. Spread between layers of. cake.

Orange Honey Filling

2 tablespoons sugar 2 tablespoons flour ½ tablespoon lemon juice ½ cup orange juice ¼ cup honey grated rind of one orange 1 egg, lightly beaten 1 tablespoon butter

Mix ingredients in top of double saucepan. Cook over hot water, stirring constantly until thickened. Cool and spread between cake layers.

Meat and Poultry

Meat and poultry recipes where honey is used as an ingredient do not generally appeal to European palates, and it is said that the reason such dishes are to be found in America is due in the main to the influence of immigrants from the East—especially China—and from Africa.

To a lesser degree Europeans are coming to relish a few meat and poultry dishes in which some form of sweetening plays a part, and there may be something in the saying:

A drop or two of Nature's sweet
Will give a better taste to meat.

However, our concern is with honey and there are a few meat and poultry recipes where the addition of this ingredient can add to the spice of life!

Baked Ham
    1 ham 1 cup honey breadcrumbs cloves crushed pineapple

Obtain a nice ham. Wipe it off with a damp cloth and remove any unsightly parts. Wrap the ham in tin-foil and put it, fat side up, in roasting pan. Bake at 300° F allowing 25-30 minutes per pound. Remove foil and skin off the rind, then press cloves in about 1" apart over the entire surface. Add honey to crushed pineapple and carefully heat. Pour resulting syrup over the ham and continue baking, basting occasionally, until a rich brown glaze is obtained and the ham is tender.

Roasted Goose
This is taken from *Recipes of All Nations* by Countess Morphy and would enhance the prestige of any gourmet's party! It is called Duaz-Fenjo.

A goose is prepared and pricked over with a skewer, then rubbed over with honey which has been flavoured with cloves, and stuffed with apples, and sugar flavoured with amber. After having been roasted (on a spit if possible) the goose is coated with icing sugar and garnished with glace cherries and almonds. The dish originated in Arabia.

Here is another which might be even more to your liking.
Djedjad-Imer combines poultry and sweetstuffs.

Prick the breast of a chicken with a skewer and rub over with honey mixed with melted butter. Pour honey, flavoured with a little benzoin gum and attar of roses, inside the bird and roast in the oven. When cooked cut the bird in half, and on each half spread finely chopped pistachio nuts, sprinkle with sugar, garnish with cherries in syrup and preserved ginger and finally pour a little more honey over the whole.

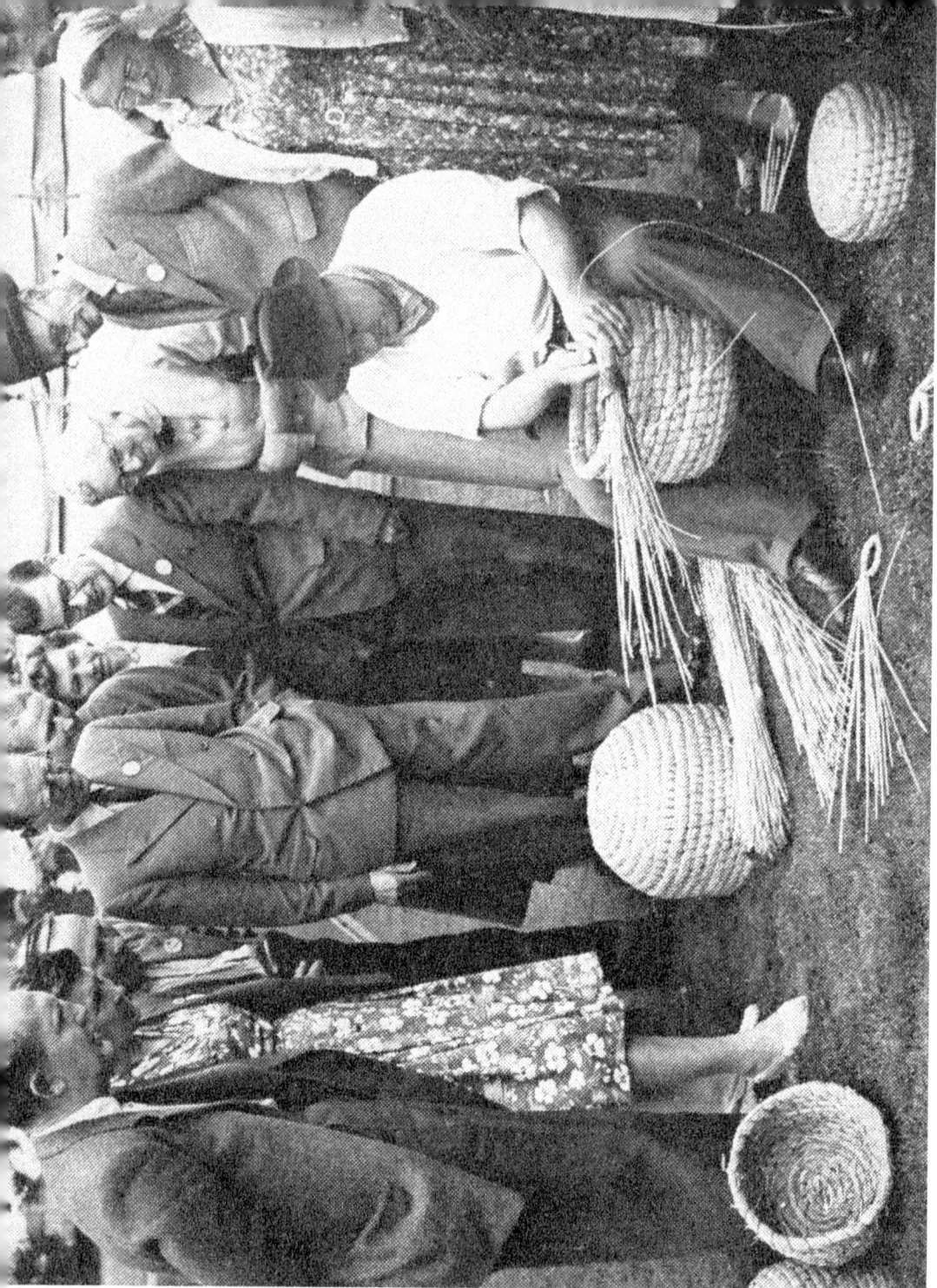

The
Skepmaker's art

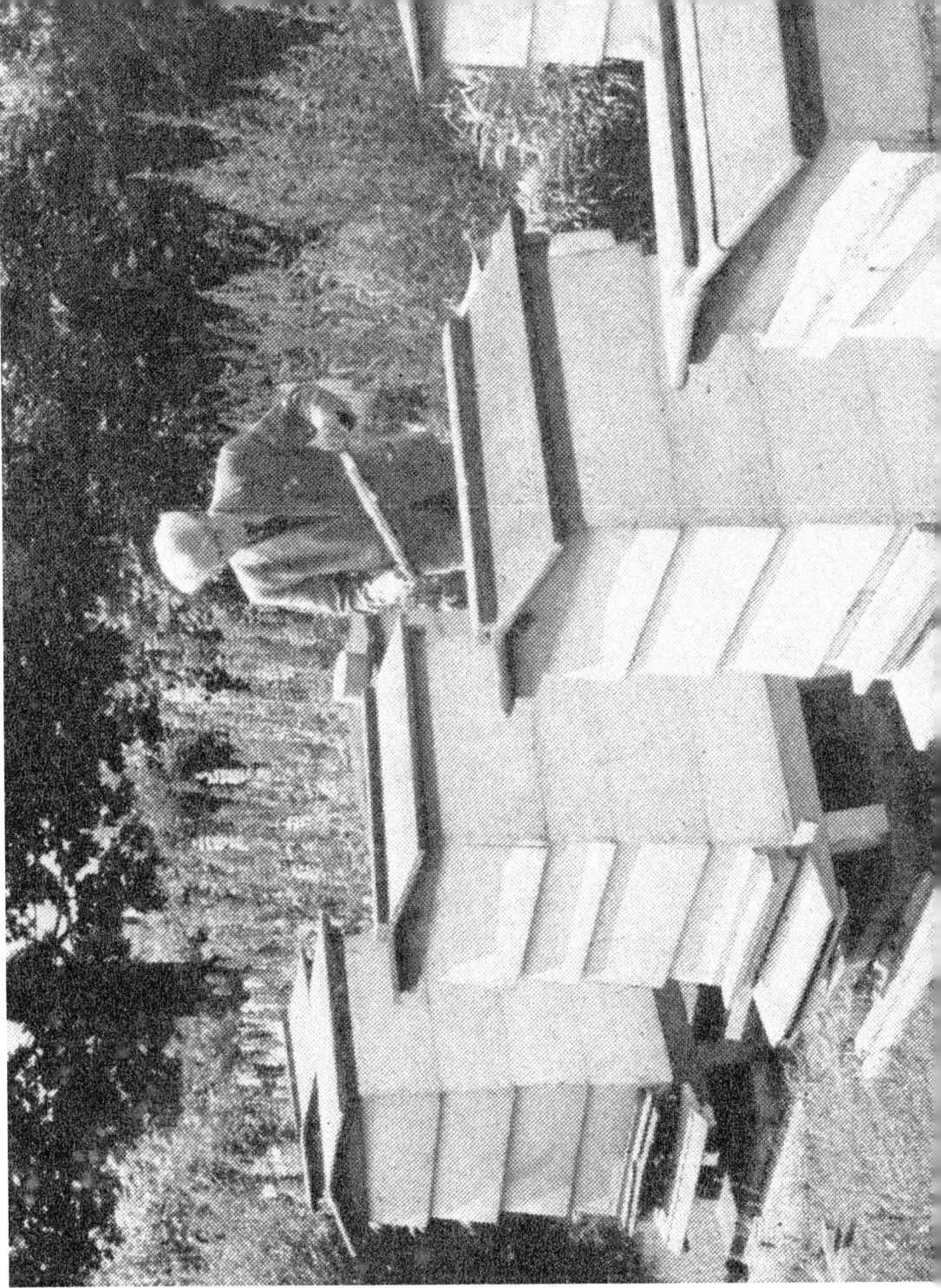

The beekeeper
in his apiary

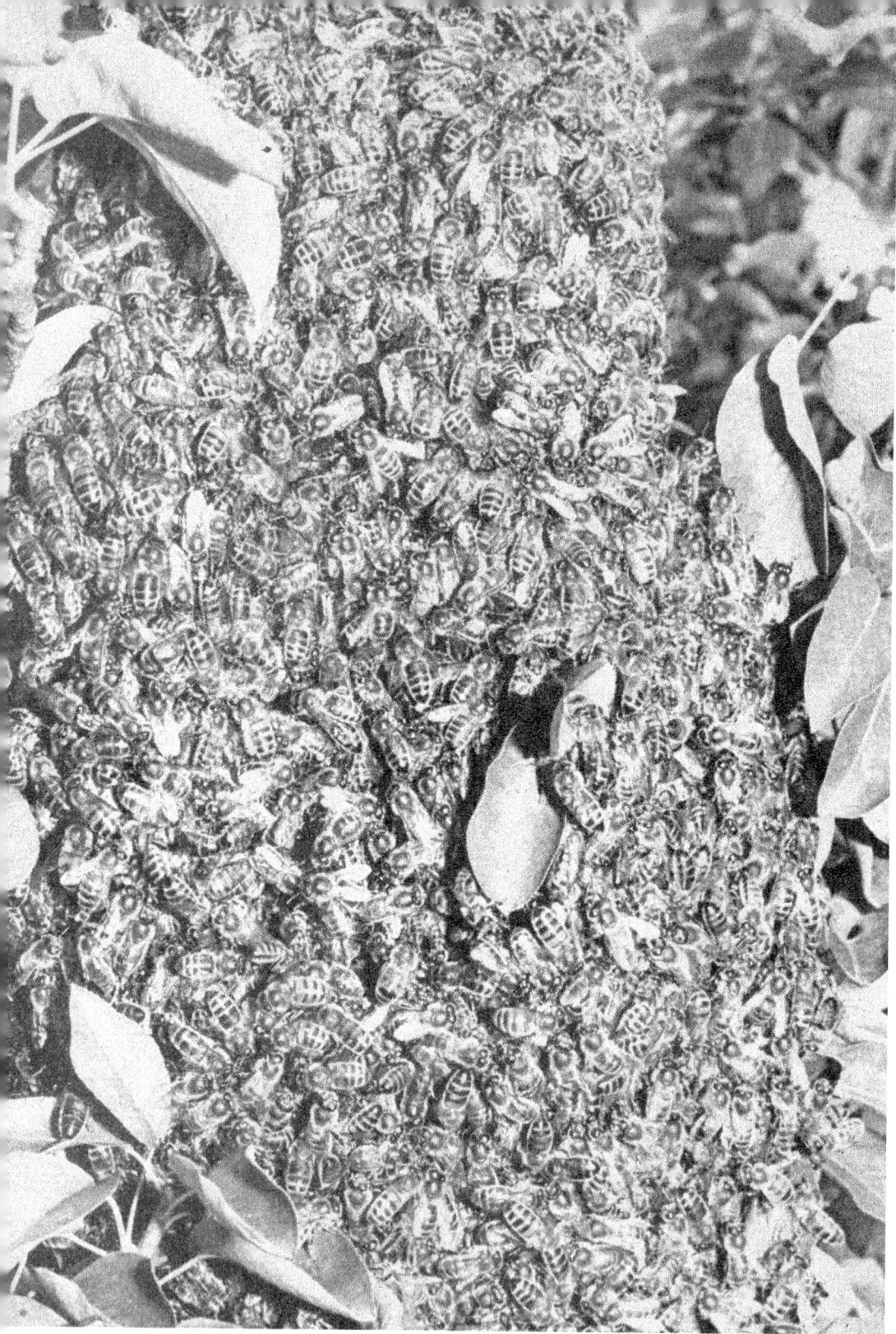

A swarm on a tree

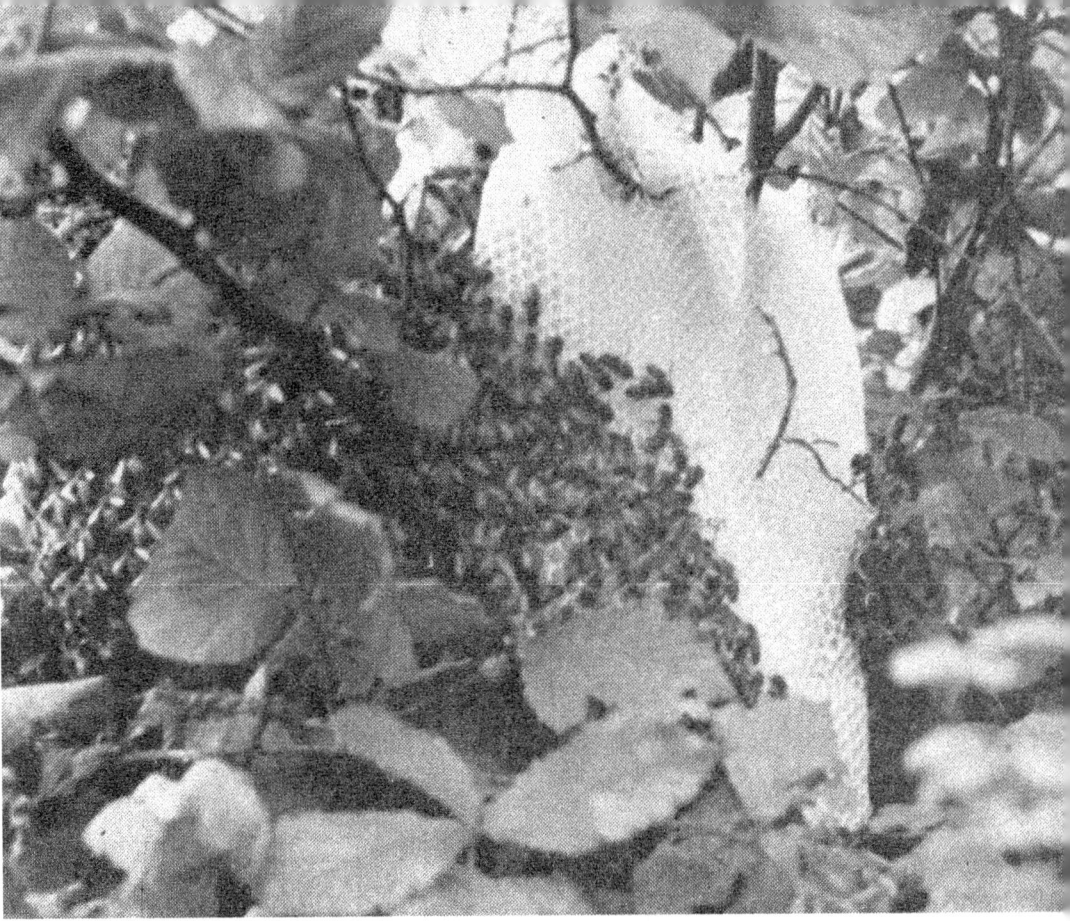

'Wild' colony in a bush

Swarming bees on a skep

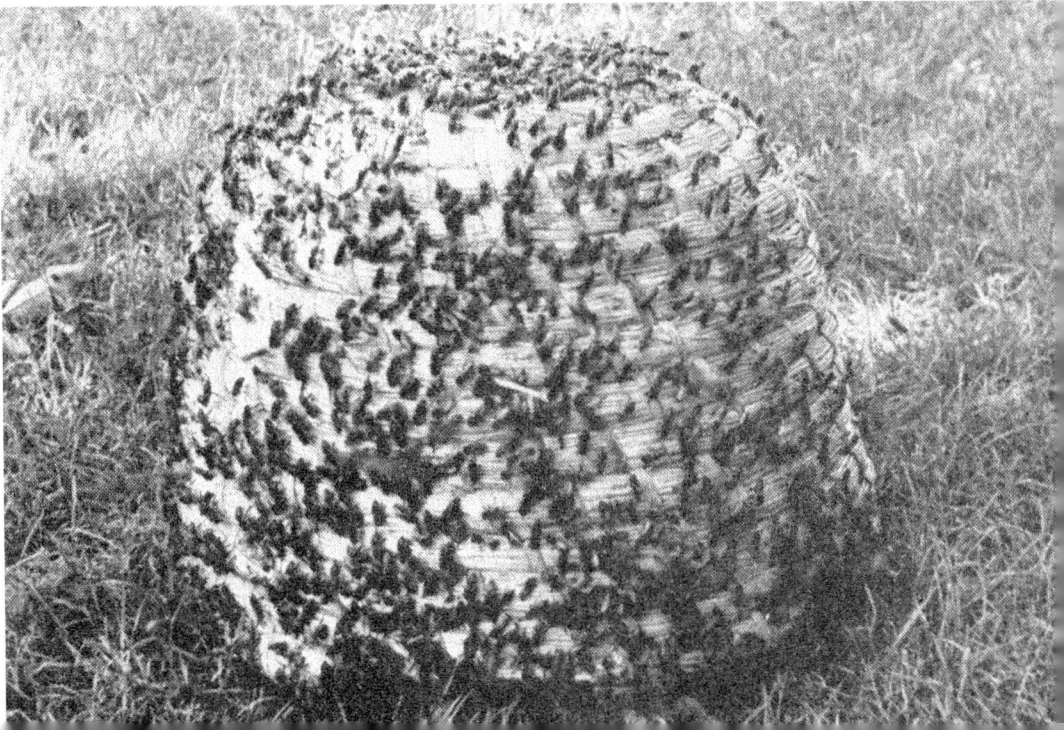

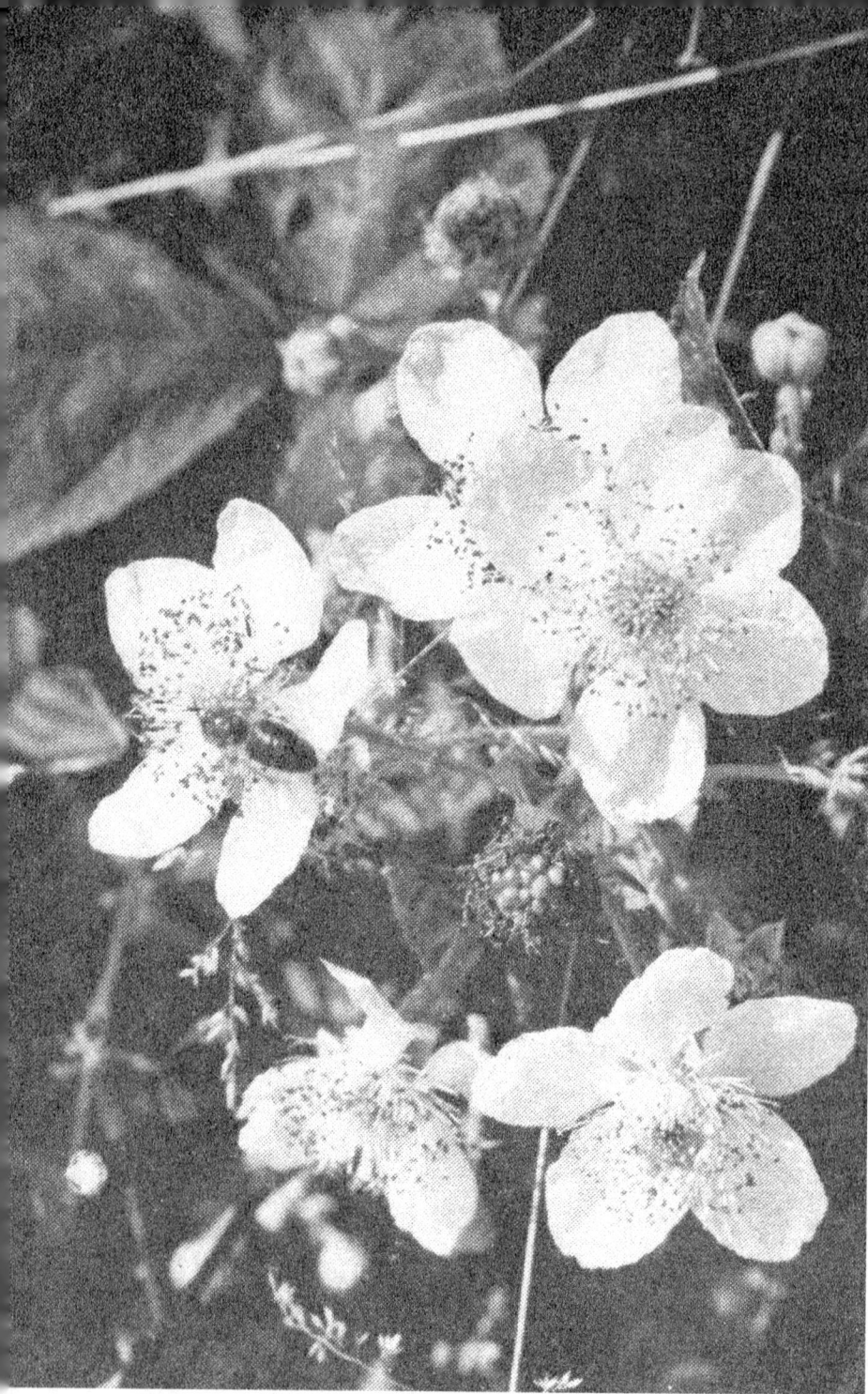

Bee on a
blackberry
blossom

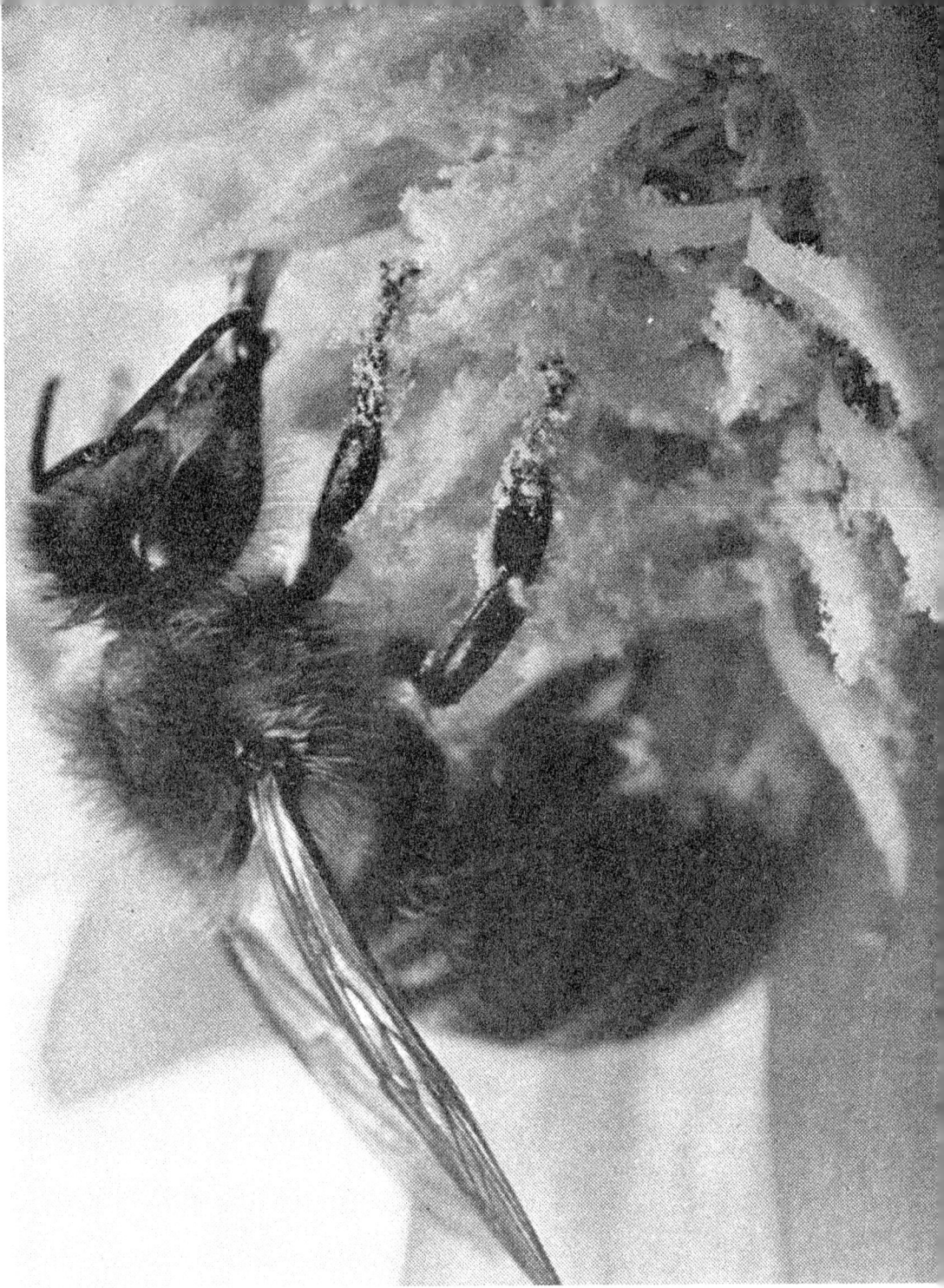

Bee collecting
nectar. Note the
pollen clinging
to its legs

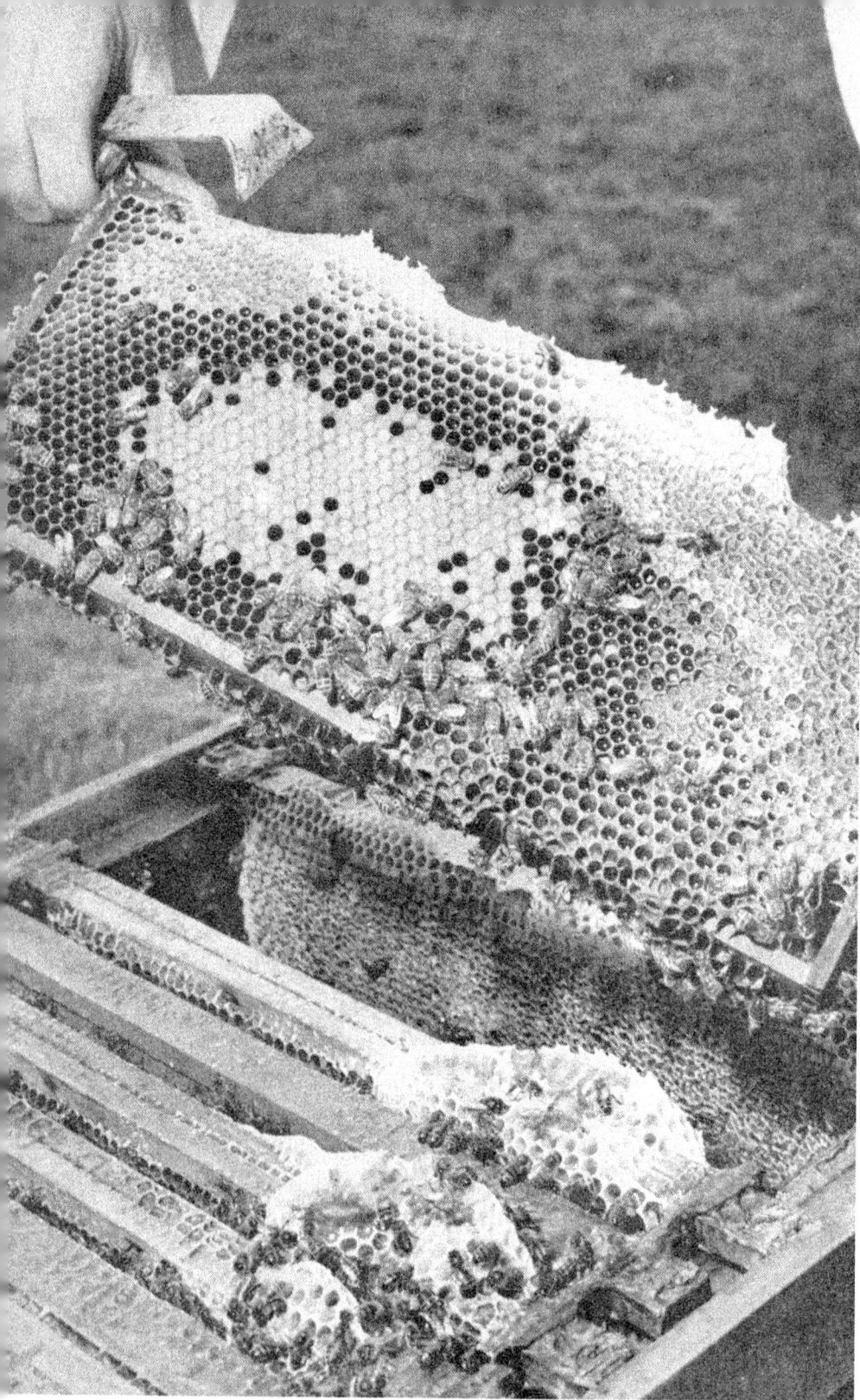

A comb of honey and brood from a hive.

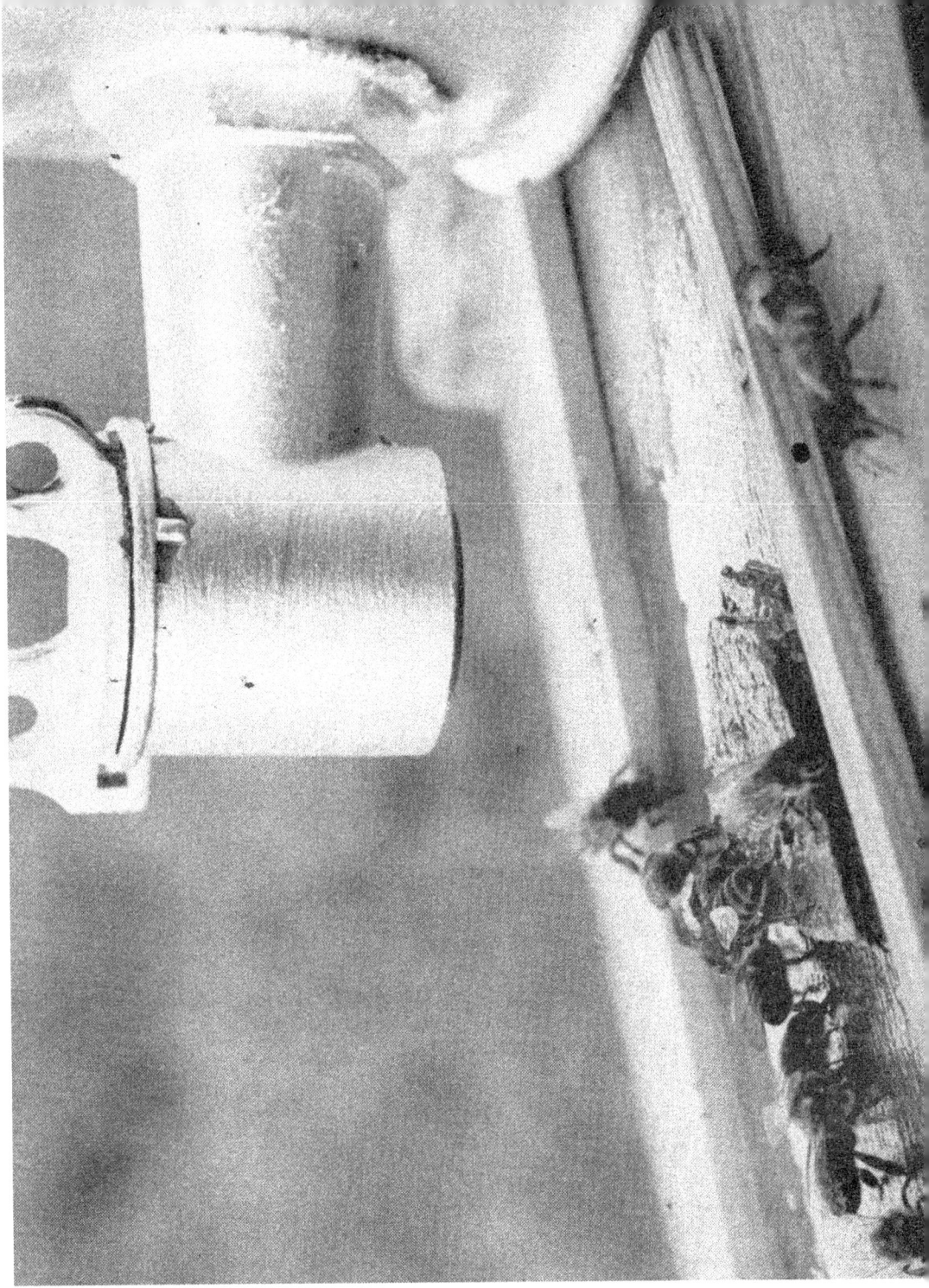

Bees drinking from an improvised fountain.

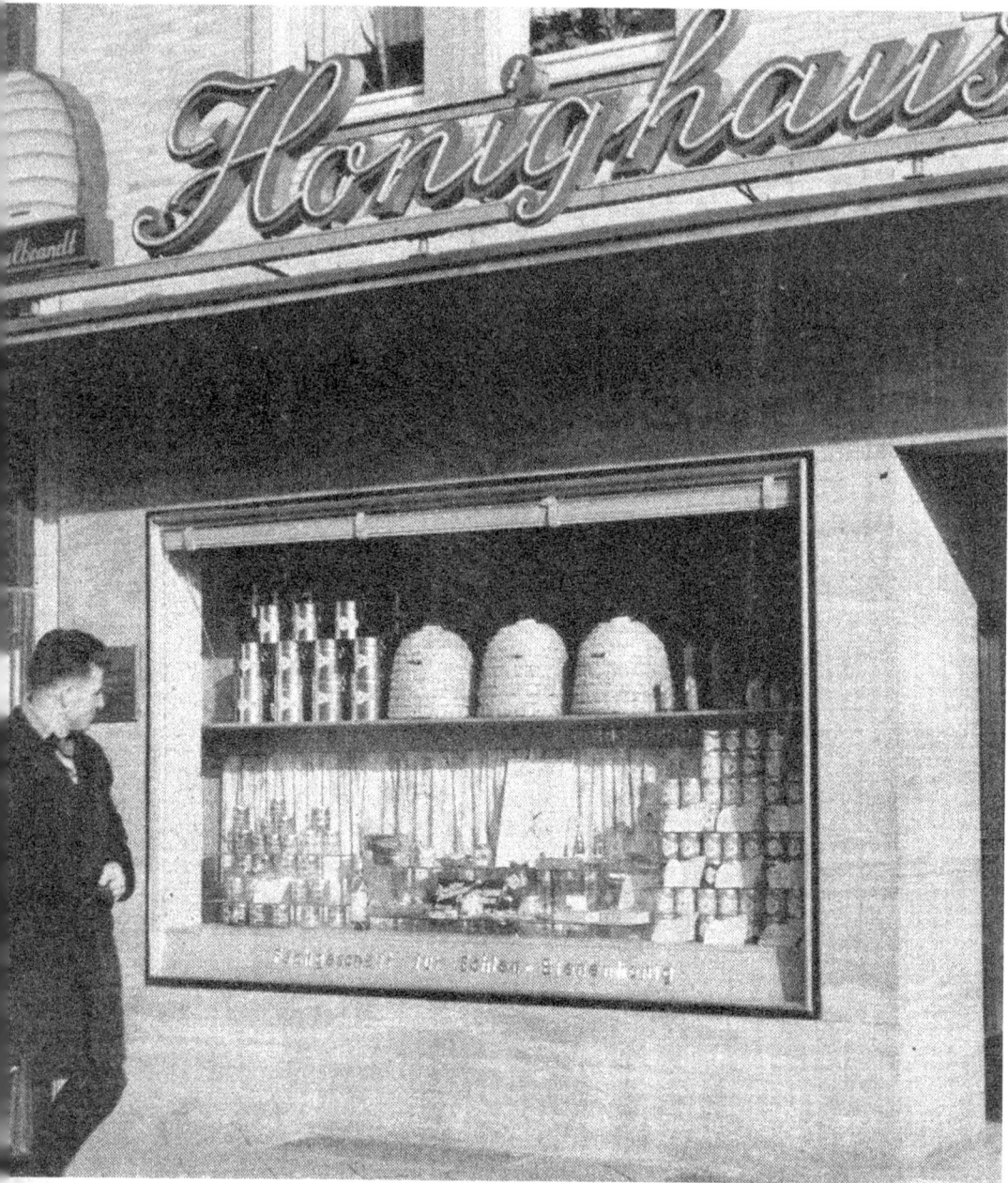

The exclusive Honey Shop in Germany.

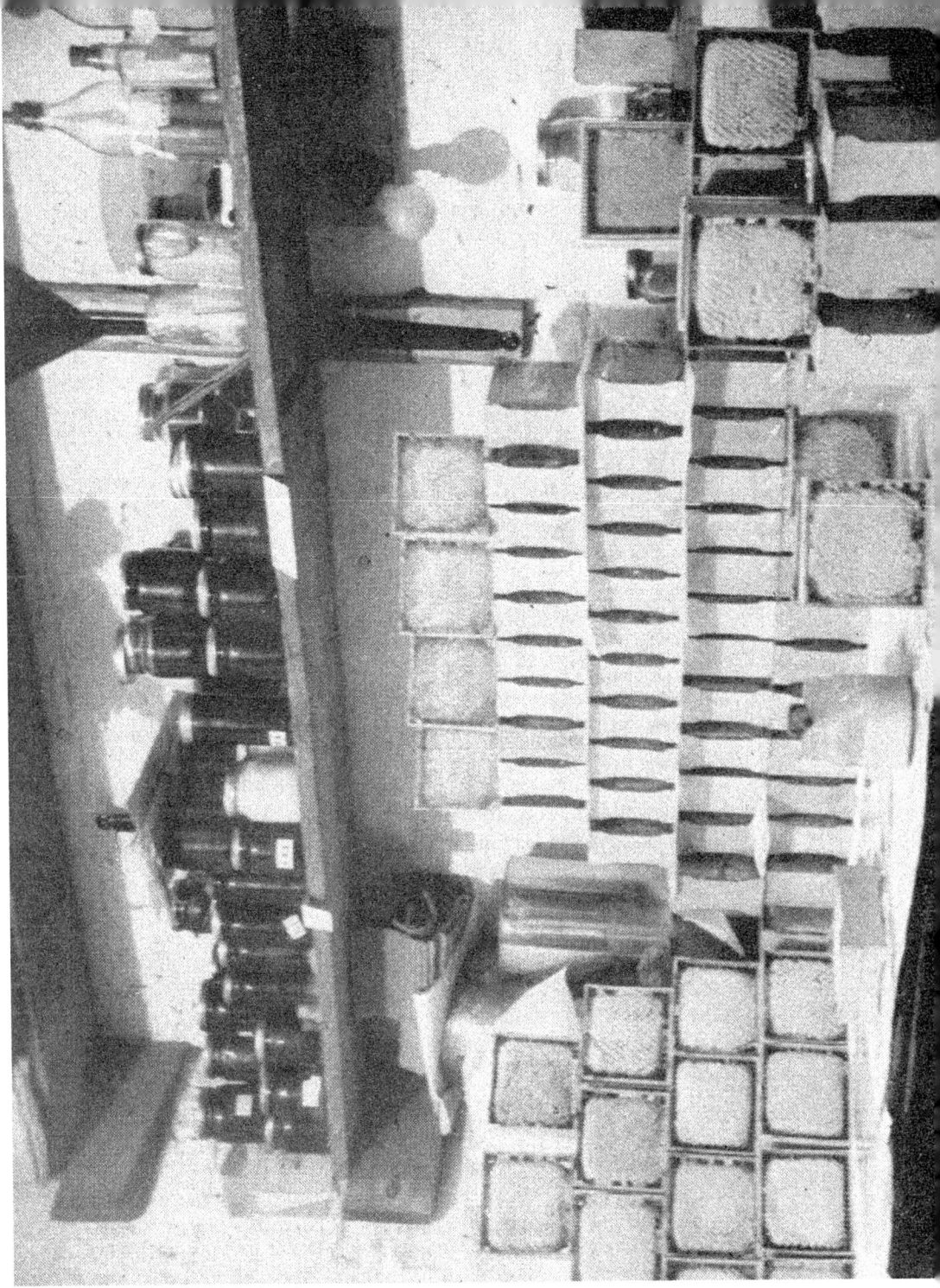

The season's
storehouse
of honey.

Glazed Chicken

frying chicken   1 egg   2 tablespoons cooking oil   2 tablespoons soy sauce
¼ cup honey   2 tablespoons lemon or pineapple juice   2 teaspoons paprika
1 teaspoon salt

Cut chicken into serving-sized pieces, arrange in greased baking dish. Beat egg, add remaining ingredients, mix well. Spoon over chicken pieces, place in moderate oven for 1 hour. During cooking time turn and baste chicken pieces frequently with honey sauce. Increase oven heat during the last 10 minutes to give pieces a crisp brown skin.

Australian Honey Board

Glazed Game Steaks

4 steaks   ½ cupful honey   1 cupful brown sugar   ½ cupful orange juice
sea salt   cayenne pepper   pineapple

Put the steaks of whatever game is preferred under the grill and cover with a mixture of honey, brown sugar and orange juice, until this becomes glazed on the steaks. Finally, carefully sprinkle with sea salt and cayenne pepper. Serve with pineapple slices.

Fine Lamb Cutlets

Lamb cutlets   milk   breadcrumbs   beaten egg   honey   water melon   sea salt
cayenne pepper grapes

Cover the cutlets in a mixture of beaten eggs, milk and honey. Roll in breadcrumbs and fry in hot fat. Sprinkle sea salt and cayenne pepper to suit on the cutlets and top with a slice of water melon and some grapes.

An interesting change to the menu!

Desserts and Puddings

Sugar figures in most dishes that may be termed desserts, puddings or sweets, so that by a little consideration beforehand and a supply of honey the sugar can quite easily be superseded.

All forms of stewed fruits, for example, can be vastly improved by the use of honey instead of sugar, and be much more beneficial healthwise.

How about a few of the following, for a change:

Broiled Grapefruit

Cut a grapefruit in half, loosen the segments as for normal serving. Sprinkle each half with honey and put them under the grill. They should be left to cook until the outer skin begins to brown. Serve hot.

Baked Apple

Select sound cooking apples, wash and remove core but leave the skin at the base intact. Fill centre with honey and one clove. Put in baking pan and surround with a honey syrup made of 1 tablespoon of honey to ½ cup of hot water. Bake at a moderately low heat until apple tissue is soft.

When using fresh grapefruit halve and segment the fruit and place a generous amount of set honey on each half as long as possible before use. If the grapefruit is to be used for breakfast prepare the fruit the night before. If dessert plates are used instead of grapefruit glasses the resulting syrup can be re-spooned on to each fruit at the time of eating.

Sliced banana with cream tastes better with a drizzle of honey on it and this is more nourishing than sugar, especially for young children.

Fruit Special
When in season, strawberries, raspberries, loganberries or blackberries can be made extra specially tasteful if they are served sprinkled with honey and dessicated or shredded fresh coconut. Preparation is best done in a large bowl and each layer of fruit sprinkled.

Honey Bread Pudding
Put three dessertspoonsful of honey in the bottom of a greased pudding basin. In another basin cream 2 ozs. of butter or margarine with 2 ozs. of sugar. Mix together 2 ozs. of breadcrumbs, 2 ozs. of flour and a pinch of bicarbonate of soda, and add these with the yolk of an egg and a little milk, if necessary, to the creamed mixture. Put all on top of the honey. Cover with a well-buttered paper and steam for 1 hour.

Honey Christmas Pudding
¼ lb. honey   ½ lb. butter   ¼ lb. brown sugar   4 eggs   ½ cup plain flour
½ teaspoon nutmeg   ½ teaspoon spice   ½ lb. breadcrumbs   1 lb. sultanas
1 lb. raisins   2 ozs. candied peel   2 ozs. almonds   1 dessertspoon brandy

Cream butter, sugar and honey together, add the eggs one at a time, and beat well. Add the sifted dry ingredients, followed by the breadcrumbs and then the fruit. Now add the brandy. Place in a well-greased basin and steam for at least 5 hours. Christmas puddings improve with keeping, of course!

Australian Honey Board

Bread and Butter Custard
2 eggs   1 pint milk   1 dessertspoon butter essence of lemon
2 tablespoons sultanas   1 dessertspoon honey   thin slices of bread

Butter the bread, cut into squares, sprinkle with fruit. Beat eggs and honey, add milk; pour over bread. Bake gently, standing dish in water, until set: about 30-40 minutes.

Australian Honey Board

Banana Cream
2 dessertspoons gelatine   1½ cups milk   ½ cup hot water   2 cups mashed
banana pulp   2 tablespoons orange juice   3 tablespoons   honey   pinch of salt

Mash bananas until a smooth cream is formed, add milk, orange juice, honey and salt. Blend thoroughly. Stir in gelatine, dissolved in hot water. Pour into mould. Serve garnished with whipped cream lightly sprinkled with nutmeg.

Australian Honey Board

Turkish Peach Cream

3 peaches 3 egg yolks 2 egg whites 1 pint milk 6 tablespoonsful honey
cherry brandy nuts or cherries to decorate

Halve the peaches and place each in a champagne glass; sprinkle with a few drops of cherry brandy. Beat together the egg yolks with the honey and add the egg whites, which have been stiffly beaten. Heat up the milk and quickly beat into the mixture. Put the bowl in another bowl of hot water and continue to beat until the cream thickens. Do not cook. Pour the cooked cream over the peaches. Decorate with almonds or cherries.

Honey Sweets

Sweet-making can be great fun, particularly where there are children, and if careful attention is paid to the advice proffered here, the results can be just as good as the bought type of confectionery. A few basic rules apply to sweetmaking:
(a) For consistent and professional finish use a sweetmaking thermometer to replace the cold-water test.
(b) Only use pans that are smooth and free from pitting.
(c) Soft sweets like fudge require to cool before being beaten.

The following terms and temperatures are useful to know when making confectionery:

Soft ball	236°-240° F
Firm ball	242°-248° F
Hard ball	250°-265° F
Brittle	270°-290° F
Very brittle	295°-310°F

Nougat

¾ cup honey 1 cup sugar ¼ teaspoon salt ½ cup water 2 egg whites
1 teaspoon flavouring ¾ cup chopped nuts

Mix honey, sugar, salt and water together over a low heat. Stir until sugar is dissolved and ingredients integrated and boiling started. Boil without stirring until temperature reaches 300° F. Pour hot syrup over the stiffly beaten egg whites, beating constantly. Add nuts and flavouring and spread on greased pan to cool. Cut into small squares.

Honey Creams

¼ cup honey 2 cups sugar 3 tablespoons water ½ tablespoon salt
1 cup well chopped nuts 1 teaspoon flavouring

Cook honey, sugar, water and salt together until soft-ball. Remove from heat, add nuts and flavouring. Beat until creamy and leave to set off on a buttered pan. Cut into pieces.

Honey Fudge

2 cups demerara sugar   1 cup evaporated milk   2 tablespoons butter   1 cup
nuts   1 square unsweetened chocolate   ¼ teaspoon salt   ¼ cup of honey

Mix sugar, chocolate, evaporated milk and salt together and boil for 5 minutes, add honey
and boil on to 236°-240° F. Add butter and then let stand until cool. Beat until creamy,
add nuts and pour on to buttered pan. Cut when set. Store in an airtight container.

Honey Caramels

2 cups sugar   2 cups honey   pinch of salt   ½ cup butter   1 cup evaporated milk

Mix sugar, honey and salt, and boil rapidly to 250° F stage, occasionally stirring. Add
the butter and evaporated milk gradually so that the mixture does not stop boiling.
Boil on to hard-ball stage (250° F) constantly stirring to prevent sticking and burning.
Pour on to buttered pan and allow to set thoroughly before cutting into small squares.
Wrap in greaseproof paper.

Cream Candy

1 cup sugar   ¼ cup cream   ¼ cup honey   1 tablespoon butter   ½ cup
chopped nuts

Combine sugar, cream and honey and cook until sugar has dissolved, add butter and
continue to boil until a very soft soft-ball stage has been reached (236° F). Remove
from heat and beat immediately. Continue beating until mixture becomes thick and
dull in appearance. Add the nuts and then turn on to a greased pan. Cut with a warm
knife when candy is cool enough.

Honey Coffee Fudge

½ lb. honey   2 lbs. granulated sugar   ¼ lb. butter   1 tin condensed milk
¼ pint fresh milk   1 tablespoon coffee essence

Mix all ingredients together and cook until 237° F stage. Remove from heat and beat
with wooden spoon until mixture thickens. Pour on to greased pans and cut into
squares. Store in an airtight tin.

Honey Fruit Pieces

Take a pound of mixed dried fruit such as prunes, figs, dates, apricots, sultanas and raisins. Clean all fruit but stand the large fruit such as prunes and apricots in boiling water
for five minutes. Put all fruit, mixed together, through a fine mincer and add a teacupful of chopped nuts. Add enough liquid honey to bind the ingredients and press mixture evenly into an 8" shallow tin which has been lined with foil or greaseproof paper.

Cover with more foil or paper and put on a weight; leave overnight. Cut into neat
pieces and, if preferred, roll in caster sugar.

Preserves

Sweet Pickle
    2 cups honey 1 cup vinegar 2 inches cinnamon stick 6 whole cloves
    quantity apples

Mix honey, vinegar, cinnamon and cloves together and bring to the boil. Have ready 3 or 4 lbs. quartered apples. Cook about a quarter of them in the syrup and handle so that they will not mash. When transparent transfer carefully to a large jar or bowl and repeat until all are cooked. Remove spices from syrup, store apples in sterilised jars, pouring remaining syrup over them. Seal jars and keep until required.

Honey Tomato Chutney
    4 lbs. tomatoes 1 lb. apples 1 lb. dates 2 lb. sultanas 1 large onion
    1 lb. honey ½ teaspoon ground cloves 1 tablespoon salt juice of 2 lemons
    ½ cup vinegar

Peel and cut up tomatoes, apples, and onions, and combine with the other ingredients. Boil for two hours. Pack into sterilised bottles and seal for future use.

Honey Currant Jelly
Clean and stem currants, put in preserving pan and mash. Put ½ cup water for every 2 quarts of fruit, bring to the boil and simmer until currants appear white. Strain through a jelly bag and measure resulting juices. For every 2 cups of juice add 3/4 cup of honey and 3/4 cup of sugar. Cook 4 cups of juice at a time and stir until sugar dissolves. Continue to cook until two drops run together and 'sheet' off spoon. Pour into hot, sterilised jars.

Honey Rhubarb Jelly
    1 cup rhubarb juice 2 tablespoons granulated pectin 1 cup of honey

Clean and cut rhubarb into 1-inch lengths, put into a preserving pan with enough water to prevent burning, cover pan and cook slowly until soft. Strain through jelly bag. Measure out juice, add required amount of pectin and stir vigorously. Then bring to the boil and continue to boil until the jelly test is obtained. Pour into sterilised jars and seal.

Additional Delights

Many and varied are the ways in which honey can be used in combination with other foods, but always remember the golden rule: use only light delicate honeys with other light delicate ingredients. The stronger honeys can be kept for more strongly flavoured ingredients.

By way of a change blend ½ lb. of butter or margarine with a couple of tablespoonfuls of Clover honey. Soften the butter or margarine by letting it stand in a warm room and then thoroughly mix in the honey until all is well blended. Pack into a glass butter dish with a close fitting cover, or a honey jar that can be screwed down. Leave it in the refrigerator to reset and always keep it in a cool place when not in use. Very good eating on biscuits or spread on flapjacks. As tastes vary a lot it is recommended that only small quantities are made at a time. The amount of honey can then be reduced or increased.

Honey cream is said to be even more delightful. It is made with three parts of clotted cream to two parts of a light honey, the honey being mixed with the cream at about 135° F. Again when the ingredients have been mixed well together they should be poured into a container that can be screwed down and then put in the refrigerator for the honey cream to firm up.

Rose Honey

Somehow the combination of roses and honey, as with cream and honey, conjures up all the delights of the countryside with its sweet fragrance. Therefore rose honey must figure in this book. To make it use the following recipe taken from Jean Gordon's *Rose Recipes*.

Bruise fresh rose petals and place a layer of the petals in a small saucepan, pour clover or a mild light honey, like Acacia, over them. Warm the whole over a low flame for two minutes. Warm to the extent that the petals may be easily strained from the honey. Pour into a jar and seal tightly. Allow to stand in a warm room for one week.

Honey Vinegar

Many of the natural products enjoyed by our ancestors have passed or are passing away in this highly mechanised, highly sophisticated, chemically-minded high-pressure society in which we live today.

The vast majority who are happy to cram themselves with the products of the machine age have little time for living and savouring the simple delights that our fathers and grandfathers enjoyed so much. One of these products is honey vinegar which, if properly made, is far superior to the ordinary kind.

The best receptacle in which to make honey vinegar is a wooden beer barrel or vinegar barrel; wood is best. Neither must be washed out before being put into use. Glazed vessels or those made of metal must not be used because the acid properties of the vinegar are likely to react on such materials and cause the liquor to become poisonous. An outside temperature of 70° to 80° F is needed to produce high-class vinegar in the shortest possible time, therefore summertime is the time to do it.

The late William and Joseph Herrod-Hempsall, great beekeepers and two of England's leading honey experts, gave the best recommendation for making honey vinegar.

Put two pounds of honey into each gallon of water (for preference use soft or rainwater). The resulting liquor should float an egg so that the shell is just below the surface but no more. Fill your barrel or vessel until it is no more than three parts full; mix the ingredients well. It is quite possible that fermentation will be set up without further attention but it is better to make sure by adding a ferment. If a small portion of vinegar plant, known as 'mother of vinegar', can be obtained, this, together with a little ordinary vinegar, should be put in the mixture to get fermentation started. Failing this a small quantity of ordinary yeast can be added to the mixture.

It is important to remember that if vinegar is used it must not be allowed to get dry, so therefore keep it submerged in liquor, neither must it be kept at a low temperature or its potency will be impaired.

The ideal place for fermenting your barrel of liquor is an open shed where the sun can shine on the barrel, but if this is not possible, out-of-doors with light protection from cold winds is the next best. Unlike mead-making, the bung-hole is left open but is covered with a piece of muslin to exclude flies and extraneous matter. In six to eight weeks, if conditions are favourable, the vinegar will be ready for use and should be strained into another barrel and allowed to settle for a week or two when it can be siphoned off into bottles, or it may be strained and bottled straight away. In either case, it will require decanting subsequently into fresh bottles to get rid of the sediment.

At first the colour is likely to be quite pale, but upon exposure to light, and in ageing, it will darken.

The vinegar plant, when once formed, should remain in the barrel. Immediately a fresh supply of honey and water can replace the previous fermentation, and can be left without further ado to go through the process of acetification.

When you've replaced ordinary vinegar by honey vinegar you will not want to return to the former.

Chinese Apple Salad
Peel 12 ozs. of cooking apples and slice very thinly. Mix the juice from an orange with 4 teaspoonfuls of honey and add a dash of brandy. Pour the mixture over the apples and garnish with a few cherries, sultanas and walnuts.

Honey Mayonnaise
The following is a good recipe for a mayonnaise dressing.

1 egg   1 teaspoon salt   2 tablespoons honey   1 teaspoon vinegar (honey vinegar for preference)   1 teaspoon mustard   6 teaspoons lemon juice   1½ cups salad oil   ¼ teaspoon pepper   a few grains of cayenne pepper

Break the egg into a bowl and add salt, honey, mustard, pepper, cayenne and vinegar. Beat thoroughly and add the oil about a tablespoonful at a time, beating thoroughly after each addition until ½ cup is added and the dressing is thick. The oil can then be added in larger quantities. When the one cup has been added put in the rest of the vinegar and the lemon juice, adding this alternately with the rest of the oil. Beat vigorously or whisk all the time during the making.

Mead and Honey Drinks

The Norsemen were great drinkers of a concoction which was something like a mead ale brewed from honey and corn and which could be quite a potent drink by all accounts. But the use of honey for making a kind of beer was in vogue before the Scandinavian countries came to adopt it, and records of mead drinking go back well into antiquity especially among the Germanic and Slavonic races of Central Europe. It would hardly have been the drink that peoples of more civilised times made from honey and called mead, but would have probably been more of a light beer. In fact there is a record that Wulstan, the traveller of the ninth century, is supposed to have told King Alfred that in Estonia there was so much honey that the king and his nobles drank mare's milk and gave the honey to the servants and the poor, who made large quantities of mead from it.

Munich in Germany has been one of Europe's largest beer-producing centres, and has had a brewing industry that stretches back through the years to the time when mead was made instead. All along the Rhine large mead-brewing industries existed at one time and honey fairs marked the festive occasions of such towns as Wurttwiberg. Along the Baltic coast and in Prussia the brewing of mead is recorded in the ancient chronicles. Local kings granted special privileges to the mead makers and no doubt were rewarded in return. Many place names in Central Europe are named from the bees, such as Bienenhof, Immichen and Zeidelwald— the latter coming from *zeideln*, to collect honey. And there is no doubt that the word 'beer' originated from a word for bee and had some early connection because honey was first used in beer-making to sweeten it.

Among the Danes and Ancient Britons mead was held in the highest esteem, probably because after quaffing large quantities of this potent liquid the old warriors would lose all sense of the world around them and their immediate worries and fall into a drunken stupor. Large quantities of mead were said to be drunk in Valhalla in the great hall of the dead heroes.

Much attention was paid to the production of mead in Tudor times, and during the reign of Elizabeth I the making of mead ranged from a simple honey-and-water-brewed ale to the most elaborate recipes calling for hops, ginger, various types of fruit and rare spices.

Elizabeth herself had her own special metheglin brewed by the monks of Anglesey island, and others were forbidden to use the recipe under the severest penalties.

To give an idea of the enormous business that must have been carried on in mead brewing here is an incident that took place at Meissen in Germany in 1015. A fire broke out in the town and being short of water at the time the inhabitants quelled the flames with the local mead.

With the advent of sugar and the popularity of wines made from the grape, and the growth of the beer industries, mead-making declined until just after the last war when a firm in Cornwall set out to repopu-larise the beverage. It did not catch on then but the growth of amateur wine-making in England gave mead its first real revival and mead-making is becoming a very popular pastime once more.

Good Health

Drinking today, of all kinds, is rather different from the kind practised by our forefathers when there was time enough to enjoy the full fragrance and goodness of natural fruits and sweetness. Today our palates are soiled by the constant outpouring of a wide variety of synthetic substances wherein only a little or none of the natural product is present.

Honey to the ancients, and even earlier to the period when Man first appreciated that natural sugars could be made into a drink with a great deal more potency than water, played a most important role in their drinking habits. Long before grapes revolutionised the wine-making business honey was the basis of many alcoholic liquors from the simple mead ales of the Norsemen to the more sophisticated beverages known as melomels, metheglins, pyment, hippbcras, and cyser, wherein a variety of herbs, spices, fruits, etc., are used in an endeavour to improve the flavour of the finished wine.

Now that there has been an enthusiastic revival of mead-making the use of some of the Elizabethan recipes, for metheglin especially, has proved that they must have been vile drinks indeed. However, there are several forms of mead that are quite excellent drinking and very health-promoting.

For those amateur winemakers who would like to tackle the subject of mead-making seriously there are now a number of excellent references and the following come to mind.

Making Mead by Bryan Acton and Peter Duncan, an Amateur Winemakers' publication, *Mead Making* by C. B. Dennis, published by the Central Association of Beekeepers; and there is a very useful section on Mead in *Amateur Wine Making* by S. M. Tritton, published by Faber and Faber.

However, as mead-making is a use for honey, and therefore justly comes within the orbit of this work, it might be of interest to give the rudimentary principles and a recipe or two for the making of mead.

Firstly, it is rather important to select honey suitable for the job and not to listen to beekeepers who, when asked about the best type of honey to use, usually say that any honey will do. From a fairly wide experience of mead-making the author has found that some honeys, such as those derived from brassicas (the cabbage family) or in places where honey-dew may be collected by the bees to mix with the normal honey of the hive, are not recommended as they often produce undesirable 'off flavours' in the finished product which is quite out of character with what one expects from a wine.

Both English or foreign honeys make excellent meads, and the best honey for a straight mead, ie. the fermentation of honey in water with a yeast, is a light-coloured uniflora honey such as Acacia, Clover, Yellow Box or Lime, although a good Orange Blossom or Tasmanian Leatherwood are useful honeys.

As honey is easily obtainable these days in single-flower variety we will assume that the potential mead maker has obtained a supply. It is also assumed that he has the necessary equipment such as a one-gallon glass jar, a fermentation lock, a length of rubber tubing, Campden tablets and a few basic ingredients to maintain a selected yeast.

The first process is to sterilise any equipment to be used in holding the 'must'. Then sterilise the honey and water. Boil the water, allow it to go off the boil for two or three minutes, and then mix in the amount of honey required.

Next squeeze the juice from two lemons, and add this to the 'must', followed by a pinch of Epsom salts, a teaspoonful of very strong tea and a ¾ teaspoonful of Marmite (these ingredients are for 1 gallon of 'must').

Put the whole of the ingredients into a glass container and lightly plug the mouth of the vessel with cotton wool. When the temperature of the 'must' has fallen to around 78° F add the yeast, according to the maker's instructions. Maury and Sauterne yeast are useful for most types of mead, although the author, on one occasion, produced a good sweet mead using a Spanish sherry yeast.

Following the first burst of fermentation an airlock must replace the cotton wool plug and thereafter remain fitted apart from racking and inspections. Keep the vessel in a warm temperature to ensure a good and constant fermentation of the 'must'.

As soon as fermentation has died down, and certainly within a few days of it finishing, carry out your first racking to a clean vessel, making sure to add a Campden tablet for every gallon. As soon as a deposit forms again, or about three months following the first racking, make a second, again adding another Campden tablet for every gallon of mead made. Further, at each racking there is going to be a little more air space in the jar containing the maturing mead. This can be made up with water, but if some extra 'must' is made up at the time of starting the bulk the former can be used for topping-up purposes.

Further rackings will be necessary at intervals of three to four months and each time one Campden tablet should be added per gallon (by the way, avoid aeration to the liquid as much as possible during racking). Drink after eighteen months to three years.

These are simple instructions for those who would venture into the realms of mead making, and the complete beginner to this fascinating hobby will, if the details are carried out carefully, produce a tolerably good mead, but for the more serious student of the art of winemaking, and one who has had some previous practice, it is better to use the correct chemicals and additives.

For those who have a knowledge of winemaking and can adjust the 'must' accordingly here are the additives for a straight mead:

> 4 gms. ammonium phosphate
> 2 gms. potassium phosphate
> 1 gm. magnesium sulphate
> 7-8 milligrams Vitamin B (half tablet)
> 2 gms. tannic acid
> 6.5 gms. tartaric acid
> 10.5 gms. malic acid
> 3.5 citric acid

Acton and Duncan in their book *Making Mead* offer some excellent advice on dealing with such small quantities of ingredients as those shown above. They suggest that it is better to purchase twenty times the weight of each additive, except the vitamin tablet which is best added separately, made up in two pints of distilled water. It is then easy enough to put two fluid ounces of the mixture to every gallon of mead made and store the rest for future use in the refrigerator where it keeps quite well.

Having provided you with the basic idea for making mead here are a couple of recipes which will be found easy to handle.

Dissolve 3 lbs. of Clover or Acacia honey in about ½ gallon of hot boiled water; add the additives and make the volume of 'must' up to one gallon. Add two Campden tablets. After 24 hours give a Maury yeast starter to the 'must' and ferment on. This should produce a good dry mead. Follow the instructions as already given for making mead.

For a sweet mead prepare the 'must' as above with 3 lbs. of Tasmanian Leatherwood, Orange Blossom honey or Clover honey. Ferment on until the gravity drops to 5 using a Sauterne yeast. Then add ¼ lb. honey per gallon of 'must' making sure that the honey is thoroughly dissolved into the bulk. When the gravity again drops to 5 add another ¼ lb. of honey per gallon. This procedure can be repeated each time the gravity drops and fermentation ceases. Then rack and follow the normal procedure.

The production of melomels, metheglins, pyments, and cysers are all variations of a theme based on the use of fruits, fruit juices, flowers, herbs, spices, etc., in mead, and for those who would like to enjoy the excitement of making and drinking these concoctions of a bygone age there is no better work than that of Acton and Duncan, who has endeavoured to streamline some of the very old recipes to make them both workable and palatable as wines.

Meanwhile the much simpler types of thirst quenchers and healthiful drinks sweetened with honey instead of granulated sugar are legion.

Every type of fruit juice can be enhanced and made to taste better with the addition of honey, and if something with a 'kick' in it is needed try lime juice, a little gin, soda water and sweeten with Acacia or Clover honey: add ice and a bit of broken borage leaf to top it off.

Honey Lemonade
1 cup honey ½ cup lemon juice 1 quart water pinch of salt

Mix honey with the water, add the lemon juice and salt. Can be served as a hot or cold drink depending upon the weather.

Fruit Punch
1 cup honey 1½ cups freshly made strong tea 1 cup orange juice 1 pint ginger ale ½ cup lemon juice 1 cup crushed fresh fruit pinch of salt

Mix together all ingredients except the ginger ale. Just before serving add ginger ale and broken ice. If too strong weaken with iced water.

Honey Mint Syrup
Boil together 6 good tablespoonfuls of finely chopped mint, a teacupful of honey, the same amount of water and half this quantity of fresh lemon juice for 10 minutes. Strain and allow to cool. For a refreshing summer drink, dilute with water to taste.

Honey and Elderberry Syrup
Strip ripe elderberries from their stalks and just cover with water. Boil for 10 minutes and then strain. For every pint of juice obtained add 6ozs. of honey and return to boil for a further 5 to 10 minutes. Skim, and bottle. Dilute with water to drink.

Edinburgh Eggnog
1 egg 1 teaspoon honey ½ cup milk ⅛ teaspoon ground ginger
⅛ teaspoon cinnamon 2 teaspoons rum or brandy

Separate egg and beat white until quite stiff. Add honey and beat in well. Beat together egg yolk, milk, spices and rum. Fold in egg white. Serve in a long glass.

The Australian Honey Board who put out the next recipe refer to it as containing 'all the goodness of the natural foods—Honey, Eggs and Milk'.

For a health-giving aid in the morning make up equal parts by volume of apple-cider vinegar and honey and store it in the refrigerator. One table-spoonful mixed in a glass of water just before breakfast is guaranteed to keep one in trim, according to the late Dr D. C. Jarvis, M.D., who studied the life history of many of the folk of his native Vermont, U.S.A., and who wrote a book on the remarkable longevity and the folk medicine of these people. In this delightful book, *Folk Medicine*, he recalls many of the simple but highly effective remedies which these people used to cure their ills and prolong their lives—and. basically, much of the treatment involved apple-cider vinegar and honey.

One or two of the following honey drinks may appeal to those who like good wholesome living.

Honey Orange Beverage with Cream
This is prepared by whipping the yolk of an egg into 6 tablespoonfuls of honey in a glass of orange juice. Mix well together and then top up with fresh cream.

Honey Strawberry Beverage
A glass and a half of fresh milk, 2 tablespoonfuls of honey and half a glass of mashed strawberries are mixed together, a pinch of salt added and the whole whipped to a uniform mass.

Honey Raspberry Beverage
Two tablespoonfuls of fresh raspberry juice and a tablespoonful of honey are added to a glass of milk, stirred together and diluted with water to taste.

Honey Cherry Beverage
Half a glass of cherry juice is mixed with a table-spoonful of lemon juice, two table-spoonfuls of honey and a pinch of salt added to the mixture, then stirred into a glass and a half of milk.

All these drinks, say the Russians, who have invented them, should be drunk cold to really appreciate their excellence. Other and equally exciting beverages can be concocted with other fruit-juice ingredients with the addition of milk.

Honey Nightcaps
Hot drinks of one kind or another, simple as a glass of hot water or as complicated as a Negus or Bishop, are principally intended to restore warmth and circulation of the blood on a cold winter's night, stimulate conversation when it might easily flag, and bring cheer to the proceedings of any party, or bring sound sleep to the recipient.

A tablespoonful of honey in a glass of hot water or milk sipped before retiring will give you healthful, restful sleep, and if drunk regularly it will benefit both those engaged in hard physical work or the elderly who find it difficult to complete a night's sleep.

However, there are other occasions when hot drinks are intended for stimulating a party, a conversation, or just as a stimulating change from the ordinary, and it is then that one usually looks to drinks like Punch or Bishops to bring the desired effect.

Unfortunately, in these more sophisticated times when the art of entertaining oneself and the rest of the company is largely taken over by prepared or piped entertainment, a glass of 'champers' or sherry is usually enough to set the seal of success on most parties. In earlier days the concoction of winter beverages was considered as important as the preparation of the food itself. As a result mixed drinks of one sort or another have often come to be named after those who invented or contrived them. Thus we have the famous Colonel Negus, an eighteenth-century M.P. for Ipswich, who compounded a hot spiced port, since when all hot drinks of this type have been dubbed neguses. Other hot winter drinks in which port wine was used were known as Bishops, but Bishops can have substitutions for port and still be interesting and stimulating.

Here, for example, is a Bishop in which honey can be incorporated which will put everybody in a good mood and send them to bed happy with the whole world.

Honey Bishop

Prick a good juicy lemon all over and insert up to 12 or so cloves in the rind. Put the lemon in the oven and slowly heat it. Into a saucepan put 1 pint of water, 4 tablespoonfuls of honey, cinnamon, mace and mixed spice, and slowly bring to the boil, simmering until the contents have been reduced to half. Now empty a bottle of dry white wine into another pan and bring to the boil. Put the roasted lemon in a large punchbowl or something similar and steadily pour the contents of the 2 saucepans in together. Add the juice of one lemon, a grate of nutmeg, a tot of brandy. Serve hot.

Harry's Mulled Ale

A close-to-bedtime beverage of Henry VH's court was made as follows:

Mix 5 dessertspoonfuls of a light or medium-coloured honey in about a pint of water, add 4 or 5 cloves and an eggspoonful of allspice and bring to the boil. In another saucepan bring to the boil 2 pints of dark ale. Blend the two together, add a tot of brandy and a slice of lemon. Drink warm.

Mulled Honey Wine

Acton and Duncan in their book *Making Mead*, give a very good recipe for making a quick mulled wine (and most people want to be quick these days, although to enjoy fully the pleasure of any wine the drinker really should be unhurried and at ease with the world).

However, for a drink on a winter's night that will satisfy try this:

Take a bottle of red or white dry wine, ¼ oz. citric acid, a teaspoonful of whatever spices happen to be handy, and a couple of cloves. Pop the lot into a saucepan and just bring to the boil. During the heating process mix in small quantities of honey until the taste is found to be satisfactory and then serve whilst still hot.

66

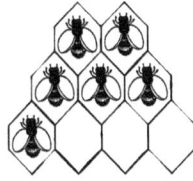

6

Honey in Medicine and Surgery

THE USE of honey as a medicine goes far back into antiquity, and even before the founding of any civilisation, when primeval man was making his first experiments into the therapeutic value of various plants and substances. And with the dawn of records the mention of honey is with reference to it being a magical food and later as a healer.

Many references are found both in mythology and in the Bible, the Koran and the Talmud to the benefits of honey in health, and often honey was an ingredient of embrocations and liniments for the cure of such irritating things as boils, carbuncles, warts and burns. Indeed, honey was frequently referred to as a remedy to cure all ills.

Honey was an important substance so far as the Jews were concerned and the Old Testament of the Bible bears witness to this. In Islam, too, the value of honey was acknowledged both as a food and for the relief of all the evils that beset Man.

St Ambrose, the patron saint of beekeepers, is reported to have said: 'the fruit of the Bees is desired of all, and is equally sweet to kings and beggars and it is not only pleasing but profitable and healthful, it sweetens their mouths, cures their wounds and convaies remedies to inward ulcers.'

Egypt is a land well-known for its beekeeping in ancient times; some of the first migratory beekeepers of the world were found on the banks of the Nile where they kept their bees on boats and moved them up and down the river following the changing seasons, thereby enabling their bees to obtain honey harvests over a much longer period than the beekeeper whose bees were confined in one place.

The *Papyrus Ebers* praises the medicinal value of honey as a medicine for both internal and external use. It recommends the use of honey in surgical dressings for both burns and ulcers and says it is good for weakness and inflammation of the eyes. The Egyptians believed that cataracts would heal from treatment by honey, which brings to mind the little story by Dr Bodag Beck of Vigerius who wrote: I have cured a Horse stone blind with Honey and Salt and a little crock of a pot mixed. In less than three daies, it hath eaten off a tough filme, and the Horse never complained after.'

In the Far East it was the custom at one time, especially among the Chinese, to 'embalm' with honey anyone suffering with smallpox because it caused the malady to clear up quickly and it also prevented the dreaded scars that this foul disease leaves.

Among the peoples of Europe honey has always found favour in the preparation of medicines and ointments. An ointment which is regularly mentioned in old country recipes and folk lore is equal parts of honey and flour mixed together. A little water can be added but the water is not necessary. Propolis—a gummy substance exuded by trees such as is found on the scales protecting the leaf-buds of horse-chestnuts in spring and collected by honey-bees to plaster up the cracks in their homes—is sometimes added. Wounds, slight or severe, skin troubles of various kinds and difficult cases of festerings, were more often than not treated with honey or a concoction in which honey figured as an ingredient.

Talking of severe wounds, here is an account of an operation given by Dr Bodeg Beck which concerns a native Indian surgeon during the building of the Panama Canal.

This fellow, who had quite a reputation, performed a disarticulation of a hip joint. Beck says he smoked cigarettes incessantly during the operation, picking them up with his bloody fingers and laying them down again. After suturing the stump he took handfuls of honey from a pail and smeared it over the wound, then covered it with gauze.

The 'surgeon' assured a Dr W. E. Aughinbaugh, who witnessed the amazing 'operation', that he had learned it from the natives of the Amazon who used ants to 'suture' extensive injuries with their strong mandibles. When the heads of the ants were cut off the mandibles remained closed and the wound was covered by honey and liquid beeswax. Results were always excellent.

Races of the Far North use cod-liver oil for healing purposes so that it has only been a further step to producing a first-class healing salve by adding honey, and this is said to be quite miraculous in its efficaciousness. A honey-cod-liver oil ointment was procurable in Germany up to the last war and may still be obtainable.

Some may well ask: 'If honey has such remarkable ability to clean and heal and renew the body in the way that has been claimed for it, why then is it not used extensively by the medical profession today?' The answer probably lies somewhere between the fact that it is a simple remedy but also rather messy, and the big business of the pharmaceutical world.

In the 29th December 1955 issue of the *British Bee Journal* appears an article by Mr Michael Bulman, M.D., M.S., F.R.C.S., F.R.C.O.G., who was at the time obstetric and gynaecological surgeon to Norfolk and Norwich Hospital; he has recently died. The article was called 'Honey as a Surgical Dressing' and it relates how Mr Bulman, after reading *Honey and Your Health* by Beck and Smedley, dropped the use of normal antiseptics and antibiotics in favour of honey, and employed honey on all his patients following operations.

The following excerpts are taken from the article to illustrate how this ancient medicament was reintroduced into the world of modern twentieth-century medical practice.

> *Antiseptic dressings involve the use of powerful chemical substances which in greater or less degree have a poisonous effect on the body tissues and, particularly when used on an extensively damaged surface, are liable to give rise to general reactions or toxic effects.*
>
> *Many different substances are, or have been since fashions change, in common use but none I have tried over a number of years have given me entirely satisfactory results. Some time ago a book* (Honey and Your Health) *came into my possession and from it I learned (page 142) that 'The external application of honey has an age-old history. The ancient Egyptians used it as a surgical dressing. The* Papyrus Ebers *recommended that wounds be covered for four days with*

linen dipped in honey and incense.' Furthermore (page 143) 'During the Middle Ages honey was extensively used in the form of ointments and plasters for boils, wounds, burns and ulcers, plain, or mixed with other ingredients.' Instances of the use of honey as a surgical dressing during recent times, mostly in Continental clinics, are also given.

Having started with a measure of scepticism on my own part and that of my staff, all those who have seen the effects of honey dressings have become convinced of their value...

My experience of the use of honey as a wound dressing has been limited almost entirely to cases of vulvectomy, usually but not always combined with dissection of the gland areas of both groins. This operation, in an area in which skin disinfection is obviously difficult, is well-known to result in a raw surface which takes months to heal completely. It has for some time been my custom to dress this surface with gauze soaked in flavine and glycerine for twenty-four hours after the operation. At the end of this time the dressing is soaked off and replaced by honey dressings which are continued, with daily replacements, until healing is so nearly complete that a plain dry dressing only is required. At an earlier stage in my use of honey I used to wait four or five days before commencing the honey dressing. I then found that by the time the honey was applied sloughing was usually well marked and it was my impression that the effects of the honey, though quite apparent in a few days, would be more rapid if the sloughing could, at least in part, be prevented by earlier application of the honey. This earlier application appears to me an advantage and I now see no reason against its use from the time of the operation.

In fact in all his later operations he applied honey after completing surgery. He goes on to say:

When dealing with a large surface it is best to use liquid honey. If granulated honey is supplied it can be liquified by careful warming. In the liquid condition it can be poured evenly over the surface to be treated or gauze may be soaked in honey and applied so as to cover the surface...

In one case of carcinoma of the breast treated by radical excision applications of honey were subsequently used on account of localised sloughing of the skin flaps. This sloughing gave rise to an area of ulceration just in front of the axilla from which the sloughs were very slow to separate. The untreated area formed a comparatively deep cavity and granulated honey was packed into this cavity daily and covered with dry gauze. From that time the cavity cleaned quickly and healing progressed much more rapidly than had previously been the case.

Finally, Mr Bulman summed up on the use of honey as a surgical dressing in the following manner:

I have every reason to think that this very simple substance provides one answer to the problem of treatment of many infected wounds. The advantages claimed for it are that it is non-irritating, non-toxic, self-sterile, bactericidal, nutritive, cheap, easily obtained, easily applied and above all, effective.

A remarkable report of scald-wounds on a man being healed by honey is given in *Alpenlandische Bienenzeitung*, February 1935 issue.

> *In the winter of 1933 I heated a boiler of about thirty-five gallons of water. When I opened the cover, it flew with great force against the ceiling. The vapour and hot water poured forth over my unprotected head, over my hands and feet. Some minutes afterwards I had violent pain and I believed I would have gone mad if my wife and my daughter had not helped me immediately. They took large pieces of linen, daubed them thickly with honey and put them on my head, neck, hands and feet. Almost instantly the pain ceased. I slept well all night and did not lose a single hair of my head. When the physician came he shook his head and said, 'How can such a thing be possible?'*

On the question of honey healing scalds, here is another which was reported in the *British Bee Journal*, 28th December 1968 issue. It concerned a young woman, Mrs Joan Marshall of Hertfordshire.

> *Several years ago, while brewing coffee for some guests on the hearth, I tipped over the whole boiling potful on to the outside of my upper thigh, unnoticed by anyone. Not wishing to break the party up and be hauled off to the out-patients, I retreated to the kitchen in considerable agony...*
>
> *I got out a pot of liquid honey and plastered it thickly over the scalded area, then wrapped and pinned a clean towel round my leg. In a few seconds the pain was gone, so I changed my wet skirt and returned to the dinner table as though nothing had happened.*
>
> *The pain had gone so completely that it wasn't until undressing later for bed that the makeshift bandage reminded me of the earlier event.*
>
> *After a sound night's sleep, I found I had a huge blister, larger than two hands could cover, but daily dressings with honey on lint and proper bandages soon healed the injury.*

Ulcerated legs from varicose veins do not often respond to normal treatment and patients, particularly elderly people, soon become despondent and debilitated. Regular daily application of honey can soon reduce the infection, leading to complete healing.

Deep flesh wounds, especially where the injury has become septic through the introduction of dirt and gravel causing serious discolouration, respond well to honey application.

On one occasion the author's son, while still at school, came off his bicycle and sustained a seriously grazed knee which would not heal easily because gravel had become buried in the flesh. After a week of no response honey on a gauze was tried, and within two days the wound was clean and healing was taking place. In less than a week the deep score marks in the flesh had reduced and finally the damaged area healed to the extent that only some redness marked the place.

On another occasion, a persistent festering had refused to heal and the poison began to work up the wrist. Honey not only opened up the wound but reduced the swelling in a matter of days leaving clean healing tissue. There is perhaps nothing very remarkable in all this when one knows that honey is naturally bactericidal as a result of its hygroscopicity, and its natural sugars and vitamins—small in quantity though they ares—promote new and healthy tissue in flesh. But over and above all this there are other factors present which are more often than not superior in healing power to the more orthodox pharmaceutical remedies available.

In the early part of 1917 a young soldier, twenty-three years of age, was invalided out of the British Army suffering from trench feet and in an acute stage, of Bright's disease.

Back in his home village in Essex he was told to rest and generally take things quietly, and that if he did this he had a reasonable chance of prolonging his life.

Miserably dejected and feeling very weak he took to lying out in the garden on sunny days, listening to the sounds of nature around him and hoping in some way that the doctors would be wrong and he would soon be well and on his feet again, while his wife went out to work to help support him and their two young children.

One warm, sunny afternoon, as he lay feeling rather more dejected than usual, he says, the air around him appeared to be filled with a very strange noise, almost as though thousands of insects were trying to break loose from a confined space. Then, he says, he was vividly aware of crowds of insects a short distance away from him milling around an old apple tree in the garden.

Fascinated he watched and the droning sound became less and less until he noted that the once large, loose circle of flying activity was getting smaller and a small dark cluster on a bough of the tree was getting larger.

Presently all became quiet, except for the normal traffic of sound, but the 'ball' on the tree had increased to the size of a rugby football which it roughly represented in shape.

As soon as he judged the situation to be safe the young man made his way across the rough patch before him until he was within a few feet of the dense cluster which now hung motionless apart from the few insects that appeared to dance around in the air above and below it. Then he realised that he was watching a swarm of bees.

Not knowing what to do he sought the help of the village store close by, where he was promptly told of an old beekeeper who lived at the other end of the village.

Having little or nothing to do and by now being rather curious about bees he went off to find the beekeeper. Presently he came upon the cottage and was told by the old lady who answered his knock that he would find the beekeeper in his apiary at the back if he cared to go round.

The beekeeper was just removing a straw hat covered with black veiling when the young man appeared but he beckoned him over and bade him join him on a wooden bench near to a number of hives from which hundreds of bees sallied forth, their tiny wings glinting in the sunlight that streaked through the dozen or so fruit trees that shaded the apiary.

The kindly old man enquired the young man's business and when he was told of the swarm admitted that it was quite likely to be his, but before pursuing the matter further he noted the pallor and unhealthy look of the person before him.

On being told the nature of the illness he said to the young man, 'Do you like honey?' 'Yes', came the reply. 'Do you think you could eat two pounds of it a week?' the old beekeeper went on. 'I think so, but where can I get two pounds of honey every week, especially as I am out of a job?'

'Well, I can supply you with honey and if you are really determined to get well you will become a beekeeper and supply your own honey.'

'How can I do that?' enquired the young man. 'By taking that swarm in your garden and putting it into a hive that I shall lend you.'

The above anecdote could have been told more briefly; more clinically, perhaps, but then the great point about it would have been lost. Needless to say the young man did become a beekeeper and in 1959 when he related this story he was sixty-five years of age, cured of his First World War complaint, had had little to complain about in all those years and had reared a nice family of healthy children. Honey, he is convinced, saved him from an early grave, and set him on the road to a normal, healthy life.

Chickenpox in the elderly can be a most unpleasant illness. A few years ago a lady beekeeper went down with the disease just as she was completing the extraction of her honey. The attack was so severe, she said, that there was hardly a place on her skin, from the soles of her feet to the top of her head, that was not covered with spots.

Remembering that she had read somewhere about the healing power of honey and feeling absolutely wretched she smeared herself all over with the honey she had just extracted; to use her own expression she 'bathed' in it. Then she covered herself with towelling and went to bed for three days. At the end of that time she felt perfectly well, and the chickenpox had subsided leaving her skin completely unblemished.

Richard Remnant in his *The History of Bees*, 1637, believed in the use of honey for aches and pains and itches, because he mentions 'admirable baths made of honey which are excellent for Aches and strong Itches'. One of his friends had 'a foul itch that he was like a Leper'.

From a large empty wine cask, known as a pipe, Remnant removed the head and having mixed together a liquor of honey and water, there being a good deal of honey present, he heated it as hot as a man could endure to stand in it, and poured it into the cask and 'caused him to stand in it up to his neck a pretty while'. This he did 'three days, one after another, and he recovered as clear as ever'.

The following account of the use of honey in healing was related by a lady before a large audience at the National Honey Show at Caxton Hall, London, in October 1968. It is almost as unbelievable as it is extraordinary but it is perfectly true.

Her old mother had to be admitted to hospital with gangrene of the foot but after examining her the doctors decided that she was not in a fit state to be operated on; an amputation operation would certainly give her very little chance of surviving the shock. The quandary then arose as to how this pressing problem could be handled because it could not be left without some immediate treatment.

It was decided to try honey and the patient's foot was literally tied in a bag of honey. To everyone's amazement and joy the honey took effect, said the daughter, and it was not very long before her mother was healed and able to leave hospital. At the time when this was reported the old lady was fit and well and had been walking on the foot for many months.

Hay Fever

When the pollen count is high during the summer, when the air becomes charged with pollen grains from the million and one plants in bloom, is the time of the year known as the hay-fever season. It is so important to know the density of pollen in the atmosphere that St Mary's Hospital, London, which specialises in allergies in people, has set up a service during the summer months to take a daily pollen count and relay it to the public by means of the daily newspapers.

Those who suffer from hay fever present a very sorry sight when attacks are frequent and severe, and it can and does prevent some people from carrying on their occupation during those periods of heavy pollen discharge.

Dr Jarvis, in his writings on Vermont folk medicine, first raised the matter of a natural treatment for anyone suffering from hay fever. He divided the disease into three classes; mild, moderately severe, and severe.

He recommended that a general treatment should consist of honey-comb cappings—the thin wax cappings which are sliced from a comb of honey before it is put into the honey extractor—being chewed once a day for one month before the hay-fever season commenced. If this is done, he said, the hay fever will not appear or will be extremely mild.

For mild hay-fever attacks the treatment should be taken once a day on alternate days. This will keep the nose open and dry. Should honey-comb or cappings not be available, two teaspoonfuls of liquid honey at each meal will achieve a similar result.

In moderately severe attacks of hay fever the patient should chew honey-comb, or cappings in honey, five times a day for two days and then reduce the dose to three times a day as long as it is required.

If treatment is followed closely there will be a drying of watery eyes in about three minutes, the nose will become unblocked in the same time and the person breathing comfortably shortly after that. A running nose or a sore throat is relieved in an incredibly short time.

For the really severe case of hay fever the sufferer needs to start treatment at least three to four months before the pollen season commences. A tablespoonful of honey (clear or liquid) or honey-comb or cappings after each meal. (Comb or cappings are better than honey.) At bedtime a tablespoonful of honey in a glass of water.

A fortnight before the onset of pollen take two teaspoonfuls of liquid honey in two teaspoonfuls of apple-cider vinegar in a glass of water, before breakfast and before retiring at night. This treatment continues during the hay-fever period. Take a teaspoonful of honey and if possible chew comb or cappings during the day to keep the nose open and dry.

The advice given by Dr Jarvis has proved very sound. Many people who previously had recourse to hay-fever 'jabs' no longer needed them when the treatment was followed conscientiously.

During 1959 the author was approached by a hairdresser who said that during part of the summer, in some years, he was quite unable to follow his trade because he suffered from very severe attacks of hay fever. He had been recommended by a friend to eat comb honey or honey-comb cappings; the friend had read Dr Jarvis' *Folk Medicine*.

At first the request was viewed with some scepticism and when the hairdresser returned for more comb honey it was treated as a bit of a joke. Nevertheless, the gentleman persisted, first with the comb honey and when that ran out. with wax cappings in honey. The treatment continued from October to the hay-fever season the following May, although nothing was seen of the sufferer from February 1960, when he purchased a large quantity of both cappings and comb honey, until the following September.

When he showed up he said he had come to renew his treatment and he was full of what had happened to him. The effect of the treatment, he said, could only be described as 'just miraculous'.

For more years than he could remember he had never known complete freedom from hay-fever attacks. Yet in 1960 he had not had a single day when he felt any of its symptoms. Of course, he told other people and soon other requests were coming in for cappings in honey or comb honey.

A health food manufacturer took a large quantity for experiments at a clinic where children were being treated for hay fever, asthma and similar allergies. It was later reported by the manufacturer, although nothing official was issued, that the results had been extremely promising. However, the treatment was eventually dropped on the grounds that it was quite impracticable; honey cappings were not procurable in the quantities that would be required—although comb honey is just as good and more easily obtained, though costlier—and in any case it was a very messy business to administer. The final part of the statement was probably the real reason for not carrying on.

Starting out with some doubts and a sceptical outlook, interest built up as more and more hay-fever sufferers said that they did get relief from their malady, in many cases complete freedom from attack.

Over many months of trial and error a number of interesting points emerged. First, it is pretty clear that treatment can follow a standard procedure for both mild and severe cases and all hay-fever sufferers should commence their comb honey and/or comb cappings in honey treatment about four months before the onset of the hay-fever season. That is, from December of the previous year to March. Over the period start by taking two ounces of comb honey or honey cappings after each meal, with apple-cider vinegar and honey morning and night, as has already been described, for one month.

During the next two months reduce the doses of comb honey or cappings to twice a day, with honey and apple-cider vinegar in the mornings only. For the month before hay fever is likely to commence return to the earlier treatment.

Results obtained from those who have followed this type of treatment have ranged from no attacks to only mild occurrences.

Treatment appears to build up an immunity in the individual during the period of no pollen, so that when loads of pollen begin to fill the atmosphere antibodies have developed in sufficient strength to ward off all but the very worst attacks, and even these will only appear in mild form.

Because the basis of hay fever is an allergy affecting individuals in a number of different ways and degrees of severity, its treatment must to some extent vary with the individual. An understanding of one's requirements can only come from experiment and experience.

In support of the author's theory that a resistance is built up through taking small quantities of cappings in honey or comb honey, in which there are small quantities of pollen of different kinds, in 1936 at El Paso in Texas there was a very heavy incidence of hay fever, brought about, it was believed, by the weeds growing in the area. The local authority became concerned and there was a public campaign against the weeds responsible.

Later, when all the evidence was sifted, among the home remedies tried that gave the best and most consistent relief was honey from the bees in the district, particularly when it could be obtained in comb which was eaten along with the honey.

Some types of asthma are also said to respond very well to treatment with comb honey and apple-cider vinegar and honey. The notable and talented actress, Miss Dora Bryan, publicly announced on television last year that she found great relief for a throat infection from consuming comb honey.

Sinusitis

Inflammation of the sinuses, or sinusitis, can be both painful and extremely depressing. In bad cases the sufferer is usually recommended to undergo a nasal operation which may bring partial relief, but in many cases does no good at all, and has even been known to worsen the condition.

The symptoms of sinusitis are blocked nasal passages, stuffiness and often severe pains in the front of the head. Because the membranes which compose the sinuses are extremely thin—something like a twenty-fifth of an inch thick—treatment is difficult.

However, it is recommended that the sufferer should chew one mouthful of honey-comb or honey cappings every hour four to six times a day. Each chewing should last fifteen minutes and what remains over in the mouth at the end of this period must be discarded.

An acute attack will subside in half a day to a day, with the nasal passages opening up and the pain gone.

Honeycomb should be chewed once a day for a week after to prevent a recurrence of the trouble.

Sinus sufferers will also find general relief if they eat honey as part of their daily diet.

Some Popular Remedies

For people suffering with hypertension lemon juice in honey is very effective. Nervous persons should take the juice of half a fresh lemon with a tablespoonful of honey diluted in a tumbler of warm water every day. This treatment helps to steady the patient and brings normal sleep. For throat infections this treatment is also good.

In cases of bad coughs, excessive hoarseness and whooping cough the following recipe is quite effective:

Peel and chop up finely one pound of onions, add two ounces of honey and three-quarters of a pound of brown sugar in two pints of water. Simmer gently over a low heat for three hours.

When the mixture is cool, bottle and cork it well. For treatment take four to six tablespoonfuls a day.

Raspberry tea and honey is a good recuperative for anyone suffering with measles and is good for erysipelas. Two or three cups a day taken warm.

A mixture of honey and blackcurrant is good for throat and chest complaints. Take one tablespoonful of blackcurrant jam, pour over it a quarter of a pint (five fluid ounces) of boiling water. Strain and add two drams powdered citric acid, three drams tincture of squills and six ounces of liquid honey. A very useful medicine.

Honey cod-liver oil emulsion can be made in the following way:

To eight ounces of good cod-liver oil add one ounce of glycerine, one ounce of essence of almonds, eight ounces of honey and five fluid ounces of lime water. Mix the ingredients well and then store tightly corked until required. A good winter standby for children.

Two cough mixtures that will be found to be inexpensive to make but most effective in most households during the bad weather.

The first consists of mixing six ounces of liquid honey with two ounces of glycerine and the juice of two lemons. Mix well together, bottle and cork firmly.

The second is made from four ounces of honey, four ounces of treacle and five fluid ounces of good quality vinegar. Put all the ingredients together and simmer over a low heat for fifteen minutes. Bottle and cork firmly when cold.

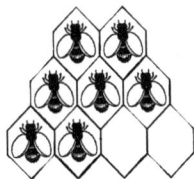

7

Honey for the Children

Occasionally, honey contains bacteria that can produce toxins in a baby's intestines, leading to infant botulism, which is a very serious illness. Don't give your child honey until they are over one year old.

IT IS a fact that honey is considered to be an important ingredient of infant diet, from a few weeks old onwards. Doctors all over the world testify to the benefit of honey in baby feeding and recommend it as a sweetening agent for milk and special baby foods. Being a natural, predigested food it is immediately assimilated into the baby's blood stream, the simple sugars giving abounding energy and nutrition at a critical stage of its growth period.

Reports from America and other parts of the world where tests have been specially carried out on infant-feeding trials, particularly in relation to diseases associated with the digestive organs and malnutrition, show that when honey is introduced into the diet, or it replaces other sugars, there is an improvement in the patient's condition.

Anaemic children given a diet of honey and milk responded well and showed a greatly improved condition over children from whose diet the honey was omitted.

Because of its bactericidal properties honey helps baby to overcome disease and because of its mild and gentle laxative property it keeps baby free of constipation.

According to Dr Bodeg Beck and Doree Smedley, in their book *Honey and Your Health*, a Dr Paul Lut-tinger, paediatrician to the Bronx Hospital, New York, found honey so beneficial to infants and sugar very often harmful, that he did not use the latter. A tea-spoonful of honey in eight ounces of barley water will stop summer diarrhoea.

Although the recommended amount is one to two ounces of honey to an eight-ounce milk feed, the mother should always consult her doctor or clinic before starting with honey.

Trials carried out in Switzerland some years ago on very young children with malnutrition and kindred diseases showed that when honey was added to their diet they not only put on weight and improved their physical condition but they also showed a decided improved mental alertness. Where children are under strain from scholastic study honey will bring renewed energy to the body and keep the brain clear and active.

A problem with many young children, of course, is bed-wetting, and parents faced with this problem experience anguish and frustration until the children grow out of the unfortunate habit. Fourteen years ago a Sister in one of London's leading children's hospitals carried out an independent investigation into the bed-wetting habits of those children who came under her care. She gave each child who showed the weakness a generous amount of honey just before it went off to sleep, also making sure that it did not get any liquid refreshment just before it settled down for the night.

Results were very encouraging and any failure was generally found, upon investigation, to come from honey that had been heated during the processing. Although outwardly the heat treatment may not have appeared to damage its hygroscopicity, when it was consumed it did not retard bed-wetting as did the unheated honey. Therefore it would be advisable to give bed-wetting children comb honey to make perfectly certain that no heat has been used during processing.

A great deal of the tooth decay today among children can be traced to the indiscriminate use of sugar and sweets, including many sweet things like sticky buns, sugar-coated cakes, and the whole gamut of sweetmeats tumbled out by the confectionery manufacturers every year.

While honey must still be classed as a sweet and a combination of sugars, being of natural origin and not artificial it contains none of the toxic properties often found in the latter. Again, being a natural product and not finely refined as most of the artificial sugars are, the consumer becomes aware of his satisfaction whereas with artificial sugars there is often an overconsumption leading to stomach disorders and damaged health.

If children were encouraged to eat fruit and honey in place of the kaleidoscopic array of sweets available to them they would benefit immeasurably and there would be a far smaller number of adolescents with dentures.

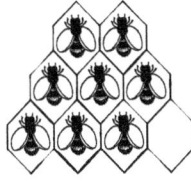

8

Honey for Beauty

THE USE of honey and beeswax in the preparation of women's beauty preparations dates back to early civilisation, and it is almost certain that such fascinating females as the Queen of Sheba and Cleopatra used ointments, salves and balms containing these products of the beehive to heighten and sustain their charm and beauty.

Today a great deal of honey and beeswax are used in the highly skilful cosmetic industry; honey because it has properties which soften and heal the skin tissue and its hygroscopical nature attracts moisture to the skin when age and the action of climatic conditions roughen and dry it, and beeswax because it is a good staple, emulsifying agent. All good lipsticks are made with a beeswax base; it is a good carrier of colour dyes.

Some years ago a young actress purchased English honey regularly in fairly large quantities from a beekeeper, and one day, when he casually remarked that he wished all his customers liked honey as much as she did, she replied that she didn't like honey all that much but every night before she retired she anointed her face after she had removed her theatre make-up. Her mother, she said, had also been an actress, and had suffered very badly from a skin infection caused by residues of make-up. One day the mother was recommended to smear honey over her face and forehead for half an hour each night and her skin trouble cleared up. The daughter was just playing safe, but the beekeeper said he had never seen a lovelier skin.

For those who would like to bring back all the pretty naturalness of youth to their skin there is a simple facial that anyone can make up.

Blend a third of a cup of finely ground oatmeal with three teaspoonfuls of liquid honey. The amount of honey is only approximate as a little more may be needed to achieve a smooth paste. Lastly blend in a teaspoonful of rose-water.

When you've got a moment to spare spread the facial evenly over the face after having first cleansed it with water to make sure it is clean.

Relax quietly with the preparation on for a good half-hour, then carefully remove it with a soft facecloth and warm water. Rinse in cold water or use an astringent. If you can use one of these facials once a week you will find that you will regain a lovely soft skin which the wind and rain may have roughened. The treatment is especially good for those with oily skins.

Queen Anne, it is said, took an extraordinary amount of care about her person and especially her hair. Her barber prepared a special hair treatment for her that was so successful that he was forbidden to let anyone know the recipe. When the queen died, however, it did become known, and it is quite simple but a very good treatment. However, it is only recommended for brunettes.

To four ounces of liquid honey add two ounces of pure olive oil and store away in a warm place such as the airing cupboard.

When you want to wash your hair, first give it the treatment. Shake the bottle so that honey and oil mix thoroughly; they will separate when standing. Then massage a generous amount of the mixture into the hair and scalp and continue to work the lotion into the scalp for some minutes. Now warm the head, say, with a hair-dryer. If you do not have one, holding your head near to the heat of a fire is quite effective— but do not get too close. Allow the lotion to remain on for twenty minutes to half-an-hour, and then wash the hair in a good soapy shampoo.

While this treatment cannot guarantee to prevent hair greying it will help it to maintain both its colour and healthy lustre, and keep the scalp very clean. Four to eight treatments a year should maintain the most difficult head of hair in good trim.

For those who suffer from chapped hands, or for the housewife who complains of roughened hands from housework, here is a good and inexpensive cold cream.

In a water-jacketted pan put six ounces of honey, four-and-a-half ounces of clean beeswax and six ounces of lard. Melt all together, remove from the heat and continue to stir until cool. Then add two drams each of attar of bergamot and attar of cloves.

For a 'quicky' for chapped hands take the white of an egg, a teaspoonful of glycerine and one ounce of liquid honey and knead them into sufficient barley flour to make a paste.

9

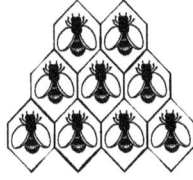

Beekeeping for Pleasure and Profit

IT IS beyond the scope of this book to offer the reader a manual on bees and how to keep them, but it has often been the case that many of those who develop a liking for honey would like to know how they may become beekeepers and produce one of the most delectable of Nature's foods for themselves. Many such people must have asked themselves: 'I like honey, what's to prevent me keeping a hive of bees?' 'Is beekeeping only the prerogative of professorial types and greybeards, or can it be undertaken by any person of normal intelligence?'

The fact that most cottages in England used to keep a skep or two of bees in their gardens for providing honey and mead shows that beekeeping was not the peculiar privilege of monks and clergy, or of scholastic gentlemen, although this class of bee-keeper has brought about the greatest changes in modern beekeeping. Beekeeping can be undertaken by any one, in any walk of life, providing they have the interest and apti-tude for it. The aptitude is the most important, otherwise interest soon wanes and some-thing which might have become a most absorbing pastime fades into a boringly painful problem for the owner of the bees and those whose help he is always likely to be seeking.

Many other questions will flood into the mind of the prospective beekeeper, such as 'How much room do I need to keep bees?' 'How much time does beekeeping take up?' 'Are bees dangerous?' 'What does it cost to start beekeeping?'

Bees can be kept in a small suburban garden just as well as on large acreages in the country. In fact some of the most successful beekeepers have had no more than a roof-top upon which to stand their hives, and at least one beekeeper obtained honey by flying his bees from a slated roof with the hive located in the attic. Bees can be kept equally well in towns as in the country, and they often obtain more honey from a town or city site. Wherever hives of bees are placed, however, it is most important that the bees do not become a hindrance or cause a nuisance to people and animals, and there must be room for the beekeeper to work comfortably whenever the necessity arises for him to inspect the hives.

For some years after the last war the author kept six to eight hives of bees on his office roof at Gough Square, just off Fleet Street, in the City of London. The bees flourished and over a period of ten years the average yield of honey per hive per year was over 70 lbs., much of it coming from the lush plant growth on the bomb sites. In October 1951 some of this honey was sent to His late Majesty King George VI during his illness.

Dr A. L. Gregg, a Harley Street specialist, and onetime President of the British Beekeepers' Association kept his bees on the narrow flat roof over his flat high above Paddington Station for many years and collected much honey. Another enthusiastic beekeeper kept his hives on his studio roof in the suburb of a large city and had excellent harvests of honey, whilst it is said that the late Lady Conan Doyle, following the death of her husband Sir Arthur, kept a hive of bees under a grand piano, and they flew from a hole in the bottom of some french windows.

On one occasion when the author was looking for 'copy' he came across a beekeeper who lived at the back of Earls Court Station, London, where only blocks of flats, Victorian houses and railway lines appeared to predominate. The 'garden' of the house consisted of a stone flagged yard approximately fifteen feet long by ten feet wide, with a few tubs of earth in which grew the most fascinating collection of exotic-hued plants. At the end of the yard rose a high wall from the other side of which one could hear the whir and whine of electric trains. At the foot of the wall, on a short bench, stood five large conical wickerwork waste-paper baskets, between the wickerwork of which was plaited straw. The baskets were inverted over short pieces of board from each of which bees flew, to circle away, high over the wall, and return laden with pollen or nectar. The beekeeper explained that he had kept the bees like this for some years, obtaining modest takes of honey which he pressed through a muslin bag. So it is not necessary to live in the wide-open spaces of the country to obtain honey, and there are some very flourishing town and city beekeepers' associations all over England.

The time that beekeeping takes up is very much dependent upon the beekeeper, but generally speaking it can be combined with most of the other activities a normal person finds himself involved with these days. The care of a single hive amounts to an hour or so per week, but again it depends upon the individual.

Beekeeping can be a great relaxation like fishing, only probably a good deal more adventurous, because bees do have a sting in their tail and they will not hesitate to use it at the right moment. Yet for all that bees are not dangerous, and if properly handled are relatively docile insects. They will generally be found to be quite accommodating too, but they resolutely refuse to be 'mastered' by even the most competent beekeeper. So it is a case of learning to work with the bees and not against them, and this can bring many hours of pleasurable interest and a worthwhile reward.

Honey-bees react to a number of things that cause them to sting. They dislike being handled roughly and will show their resentment quite quickly. They cannot tolerate certain odours, even those that may not be considered unpleasant to a human being. Highly scented clothes or hair will bring a brisk reaction. Likewise a wind blowing into the hive, or when bees are hungry. There are also right times and wrong times to inspect the hives and the beekeeper soon learns when and when not to interfere.

A prospective beekeeper may naturally ask: 'How much honey am I likely to get from a hive of bees each year?' The answer simply is: It will depend upon many factors, and as with some other natural products much will depend upon the weather and the location of the bees. Bees can generally reckon to do reasonably well year after year in and around towns and cities because of the parks and gardens and a variety of wasteland where plants and trees are grown to beautify the surrounding area, whereas out in the country where modern farming is concerned with making a living and a high cash return, large tracts of corn and barley will provide little or no return for the bee. However, if the weather in June and July is reasonable the country beekeeper may bring home a very good harvest from specially sown crops like field beans, mustard and rape, and the white clover in the pastures. Bees forage over a distance of from one to one-and-a-half miles in search of food and, provided the area is not over-populated with hives of bees and the weather is kind, it is surprising what an unpromising looking area may hold.

Before venturing further most people like to know how much a hobby is likely to set them back financially, even though any figuring can, like most hobbies, only be very tentative.

For anyone starting beekeeping and wanting new equipment and bees the cost would be approximately £25 to £30 (this in 1969 - in 2020 more like £300) For this you would get a choice of one of the several hives made, complete with all the 'furnishings' and two chambers, called supers, in which you would collect your honey. You also get the most essential tools of the business of beekeeping: a smoker, which in simple terms is a tin fire-box fitted with a nozzle mounted on a bellows, and in which a number of combustible materials can be burned—this is the instrument with which you will subdue your bees when you want to examine the inside of their hive; a net or wire veil which every beginner should wear over the face to give protection; a pair of special fine leather gloves, which can be worn in the early stages of learning the craft, although most beekeepers discard them later on, while always retaining them near at hand in case the occasion should arise; and a metal spatula turned over at one end, called a hive tool, with which to ease up the various chambers comprising the hive, or the combs in the hive.

Here, then, is what might be termed a beginner's outfit, less the bees, which we will deal with a little later on.

Of course, as with other hobbies and when acquiring a camera, fishing tackle, etc., there are ways and means of starting on a cheaper basis: there is always the second-hand dealers' market. Beekeepers sell and buy bees and equipment among themselves and use the beekeeping journals and associations to advertise their wares, but sometimes, like that secondhand car, a deal misfires and the novice beekeeper hasn't so much a cheap buy as an expensive deal.

Having decided that this is your line of country and an investment of £20 to £30 (£300) is going to bring you a great deal of healthy pleasure and a good return, what must be the next step?

Firstly, it is important to make contact with people who are already in the craft. This can be done in a number of ways; by joining a beekeepers' association, taking up a journal dealing with beekeeping, or finding out the name of a firm making beehives, etc. The easiest way is to search the internet for information. Thornes, Paynes, Maisemore, National and others all make hives. Getting hold of the local beekeeping association is not so hard. Your library will probably be able to help you or failing that, for the UK, you can visit *www. bbka.org.uk*. In Britain there are many national and regional magazines for example *Bee Craft* and *The Beekeepers Quarterly* while Scotland is served by *The Scottish Beekeeper* and Ireland by *An Beachaire*.

And in America the two leading beekeeping papers are *American Bee Journal*, Hamilton, Illinois, and *Bee Culture*, Medina, Ohio. The journals will acquaint you with the name of your nearest beekeeping manufacturer or stockist. He is usually a very knowledgeable person on bees and the beekeeping equipment you will require to set you up.

Finally, in this connection it is important to mention other reading matter. Whichever way you start, or whatever you are told or think, you should obtain a good practical manual on the subject of beekeeping. Practical experience in the main counts in all things, but in beekeeping a book knowledge combined with the practical is of tremendous advantage. Here the secretary of the association you join will know the best bee manual currently available.

You are now well on the way to becoming committed. What time is it best to commence? Most people would say: In the spring so that you have the first season before you. But really it does not matter when the plunge is taken. If it is the autumn or winter there will be no bees, but what better time to learn something about bees from attending lectures, film shows, etc. You will be ready to lend a hand when you do get your bees. Late spring is the time to get the bees and if you already know something about them and have your hive ready it is a comparatively simple matter to house them when they arrive.

A four- to six-comb colony will be sent to you either by rail or road transport, or you may prefer to go to the buyer and see your bees packed. A number of people do this and get immense interest and satisfaction from seeing the expert at work. Whichever way it is done, the little colony comprising a queen bee, a large number of worker bees and perhaps some drones on combs of brood and honey, will travel to your apiary in a special ventilated travelling box (the term 'brood' refers to the small larvae or baby bees un-hatched).

When they arrive you should set them down beside the hive they are going to occupy but shade them from any strong sunlight. In the box you will find a little doorway; this is opened to let the bees fly and become accustomed to their new surroundings. This first flight is best given in the evening just before dusk when the occupants of the box will not venture far but will spend the time orientating themselves to their new home. Next day, with the help of an experienced beekeeper, you will be able to see your bees really well for the first time as they are transferred to their permanent quarters.

The queen, if she is found, you will notice is much larger than her workers, rather slender in body and elegant in manner. She will be attended by a small group of workers who make a circle around her constantly, offering her food, and continually 'grooming' her.

The great mass of bees will be the workers, probably 15,000 or more in number. They are female by nature but unable to lay fertile eggs from which other workers will emerge; this is the sole duty of the queen. Their duties are varied and many. The younger ones are the nurse bees and they look after the young larvae in their cells, and feed them, cleaning out the cells when an occupant has emerged as a fully grown bee. They produce and construct comb, and repair comb that is old or damaged. They scavenge and keep the hive clean, help provide the ventilating system, evaporate the water from incoming fresh nectar and even take it from the older bees to deposit it in the comb during rush periods. When they are more mature they become guards on the door and repel strangers and finally, when old enough, they sally forth as foragers to provide the colony with honey, pollen and water. Their lives in summer are shortened to about eight weeks or so through continuous activity, while they may live as many months in autumn and winter when all is quiet.

The drones are the males of the colony, much larger than the workers but smaller than the queen, and recognised by their squat, bumbling appearance. They are also recognisable by the smallness of their numbers; there will be 200 to 300 in a full hive. The drone has no sting and is quite harmless. He appears to have nothing to do in the labour of the hive and spends a good deal of his time on fine days speeding from the hive in search of queen bees with whom he may mate. Nature in her lavishness provides far more drones than will ever find mates, so that his days usually pass in eating and comfortable living until there is a cessation of food supplies. Then the workers put him to death by casting him out of the hive to die of cold and starvation since he cannot fend for himself.

Beekeeping is a lifetime of fascinating study and when you think you have learnt it all you will suddenly be conscious that you are still at the beginning, and your interest will be roused again and again. You will discover that there are various races of honey-bee although the Italian and Caucasian races tend to be most prominent over the western world. However, if they are left to settle down each strain of bees, of which there are hundreds, tends to become localised in their habits and attuned to their environment. This is a good reason for buying bees near at hand if you can, rather than from another locality.

In locating your hive certain care should be taken, although bees are very accommodating. Nevertheless, for the best results a few rules should be followed:

When bees are left to their own devices they choose a situation where there is some shade and where the cold wind cannot penetrate; more often than not this is a hollow tree. In choosing your site remember this and do not put the colony in a sun-trap where baking conditions on a hot day will cause the bees to have to fan for their very lives when they should be out foraging among the flowers. Likewise do not put them in a place exposed to a lot of wind; bees hate wind. However, contrary to what is often taught the hive does not necessarily have to face south or south-eastwards, so long as it is not directly facing a right of way used by people or animals. If for some reason people will be passing across the flight-path of the bees, then erect a fence or hedge to throw the bees up in their flight and over the heads of passers-by. Avoid a spot where offensive smells will irritate the bees so that they will vent their spite on people and animals. Such places are near manure heaps, pig-styes, etc. Try to avoid places where animals roam, but if you want to keep your bees in a field with other livestock make certain the area occupied as an apiary is well fenced in.

If you want to keep bees in your garden and neighbours are close by, remember that not everyone is interested in your hobby, however fascinating you may find it. Live and let live! If possible, do not choose the time when your neighbour is out in his garden with his family, to examine the inside of the hive, and handle the bees only on suitable days. Try to locate the hive or hives as far away from your neighbour's normal garden activities as possible. Washing often gets 'punished' on washing day if bees are located too close.

They appear to be attracted to it for some reason and shed their faeces upon it, especially the whites.

Even if you do not have to do it a pot of delicious honey straight from the beehives is a most neighbourly gift that the beekeeper can bestow, and in time of tension the most soothing of salves. If it is made an annual event you will be surprised what sweet neighbours you have!

Remember that bees dislike certain odours, so on a hot stifling day when you feel damp with perspiration, have a wash in cold water before attending to the bees. Freshen up the face and hands especially. A piece of beekeeping equipment which few if any manuals on bees mention, is a fine water-spray, the plastic type that folk buy for very light household duties or for applying insecticides to rose trees, etc. If, after the smoker has subdued the bees, a few drifts of fine misty spray are passed lightly over the top of the combs in the hive, the bees will remain quite quiet and still, and those that have perhaps been running a little nervously hither and thither will retreat between the combs to join their companions. The spray does not frighten them so much as give them the feeling that rain is beginning to fall and the best place is in the hive. The water also cools the atmosphere of the hive, causing the bees to cluster.

Those Non-sugar-Fed Bees

It is as good a place as any to refer here to the unfortunate phrase that has grown up in the health food trade: non-sugar-fed bees.

What is really meant is this: any honey procured from bees that have been fed artificial white sugar or sugar syrup is suspect as there is sure to be some sugar syrup in the honey. Furthermore, bees that have been fed sugar will be constitutionally poorer than those reared and fed on good wholesome honey. Let us put it this way, those bees reared on the artificial product are not likely to be so good or strong as those able to get pure honey, but if the amount of sugar fed to a colony of bees is only to supplement their normal diet of pollen and honey then no great harm is done.

Honey-bees have lived and thrived for hundreds of years on this kind of diet given to them by the beekeeper and they would show signs of deterioration only if the sugar became their sole food, but not in the quantity it is usually offered to them. Furthermore, any white sugar, i.e. sucrose, is immediately converted by them in much the same way as they would deal with nectar or cane sugar from the flowers.

Some well-meaning folk suggest that it is far better to give the bees supplies of honey instead of sugar when their stores are inadequate or run low, but the really experienced beekeeper will tell you that this is both a difficult and a dangerous practice.

Firstly, the smell of honey is very attractive to bees generally, and when it is necessary to feed bees it is usually at a time when flowers from which the bees can gather nectar are scarce. Therefore other bees, aware of the odour and the sound of activity in the hive of the colony being fed, soon arrive to join in the feast. Soon the peaceful hum of the apiary is turned into one of frenzied turmoil as marauders attempt to get at the prize and the defenders try to turn them away. Fierce battles take place and it is not long before the bodies of hundreds of dead bees lie around the threshold of the hive. Even if the attackers are eventually beaten off, the colony will certainly be left in bad shape. This is called 'robbing' and if it should break out in an apiary it is ugly to see. Therefore honey feeding should be avoided.

The dangerous part comes from passing disease to a colony and this can so easily done from feeding foreign honey or honey from sources unknown. Even if robbing does not break out certain diseases which can be introduced in a dormant stage in honey can have disastrous effects upon an apiary. And having introduced perhaps a discordant note about disease let it be clearly understood that this kind of disease is quite harmless to human beings.

In the majority of cases bees need to be fed at some time, the most usual being autumn when the colony is made ready for winter, and often in those early spring days just before there is sufficient blossom to take care of the bees' needs. These are the most crucial times. However, the amount of food given is usually quite small when one compares it with the amount of honey used by an average colony during the season. Estimates vary, but it is somewhere between 150 lbs. and 220 lbs.

When your bees first come you will be wanting to have a look at them every day to see if they are going along alright, but if their combs are continually pulled apart they will not thrive. It is better in the early stages of your great curiosity to obtain what is known as a glass quilt which you can peer through to watch the bees at work. You will also get tremendous interest from watching the bees at the entrance; the pollen carriers with their great baggy 'trousers' of different coloured pollens; the nectar collectors hurrying without halt to get rid of their loads, while the guards move slowly to and fro among the frenzied fanners as they control the temperature inside, examining any would-be intruder and expelling it unceremoniously should it be found. Here and there will also be seen one bee 'conversing' with another as they gently rub antennae together, or an entrance guard relieving a comrade of a heavy load.

When you get more proficient the entrance 'goings-on' will tell you a great deal of what is happening within the hive and then you will know that at last you are becoming a knowledgeable beekeeper.

www.ingramcontent.com/pod-product-compliance
Lightning Source LLC
Chambersburg PA
CBHW080053280326
41934CB00014B/3307